Superior Nutrition

by

Herbert M. Shelton

AUTHOR O

FASTING CAN SAVE YOUR LIFE
FASTING FOR THE RENEWAL OF LIFE
THE SCIENCE AND FINE ART OF FASTING
HEALTH FOR THE MILLIONS
GETTING WELL
HEALTH FOR ALL
AN INTRODUCTION TO NATURAL HYGIENE
SYPHILIS: WEREWOLF OF MEDICINE
LIVING LIFE TO LIVE IT LONGER
EXERCISE
FOOD COMBINING MADE EASY
THE HYGIENIC CARE OF CHILDREN
ETC., ETC.

PUBLISHED BY
WILLOW PUBLISHING, INC.
SAN ANTONIO, TEXAS

Fifteenth Printing - 1994

DEDICATION

To my patients, whose repeated questions have revealed the great need for a book such as this one, in the hope that both they and all of my other readers may profit by the vital information herein contained, this book is affectionately dedicated, by

—THE AUTHOR

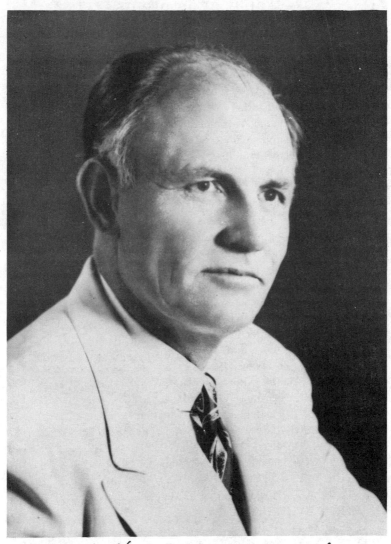

Yours for Health Truth and Medical Liberty
Herbert M. Shelton

Table of Contents

Introduction

In the middle of the last century it was stated that one-fourth of all children born alive died before reaching their seventh year, and one half before reaching the age of seventeen. Only six persons in a hundred reached the age of sixty-five, while hardly more than one in ten thousand reached the century mark. These deplorable facts were true of the more advanced countries, where records were kept. They were (and are) certainly much worse in the more backward parts of the world.

Those of us who have been brought up in America and have not been outside the boundaries of our own country, tend to think of the world as advanced. We do not realize that the Stone Age still persists in large sections of the earth, that there is savagery, barbarism, medievalism, human (chattel) slavery, etc., in the earth. When you consider that a child born of the "colored" races (black, brown, yellow) has only a one-to-four chance of ever learning to read and is almost certain not to have a radio, so that it will be shut off from what is going on in the world, you get some idea of the lamentable ignorance that exists in the world and of the reason for the survival of ancient superstitions. If you consider that it was only yester-year that your own great grand-parents were in the same state of ignorance and that they bequeathed to you a great store of superstition, from which the advance of knowledge has only partially emancipated you, you will not be inclined to boast of your "superiority" over the rest of the world.

I heard a man, who had probably never been to the South Seas, say that he could take you to the South Seas and show you men ninety years old who are as lively as young men of twenty in this country. We continue to hear of the remarkable health and development and of the advanced ages attained by the backward peoples of the earth. If you want to find men who live to be two hundred, three hundred, four hundred or more years old, you go to the people who have no calenders and no records of their births. If you want to find really old men, you go to Tibet, where the land is so filthy and the people so poverty stricken that their average life-span is probably not over eighteen years. The cities and towns in Tibet are so very insanitary that one wonders how any people can live in them, while the smell of cow dung is an insult to the nostrils of all who have not been brought up amid its stench and thus become inured to it. It is here that men are reported to live beyond a thousand years. Here, too, amid the grossest ignorance, we are told there live men who so far surpass in knowledge, the most highly educated men in civilization, as to make these educated men appear totally unlearned. They are particularly "spiritually" *advanced*—all backward peoples compensate for their failure to advance by priding themselves upon their "spiritual superiority". A young Hindu student, who assured me that he could easily see his former Master in India and converse with him across the thousands of miles that separated them, but who came to America to study engineering, assured me that India is several thousand years ahead of America—"spiritually".

Holy men in India manifest their great "spiritual" advancement, by rubbing cow dung in their hair, by hanging for long periods head down, by crawling on their bellies for hundreds or thousands of miles, by slowly and painfully trudging across the country, from ocean to ocean, weighted down with huge chains, and by other equally useless, wasteful and body-destroying practices—follies born of the dogma of the worthlessness of terrestrial life. If this is "spirituality", may the good God save America from ever making any "spiritual" advancement. Let us remain sane.

We read the glowing accounts of the beautiful specimens of manhood and womanhood to be found among the peoples of some part of the earth and then we go to the movies and see a travel picture showing actual pictures of great numbers of these very people and are shocked to find that they are no better, perhaps no worse, than the miserable specimens that we produce in our ant hives that we call cities.

We are not bound to accept the glowing and enthusiastic accounts of the healthfulness of the backward peoples of the earth in contrast to our own health. Good health among savages and the less advanced portions of mankind is spotty. For the most part, these backward peoples are sick and short lived. Malaria, intestinal parasites, tuberculosis, leprosy, malnutrition and a host of other complaints are common among them. Famines are common and hunger is a more or less constant state.

Great portions of the human family today live in mud huts, with dirt floors, thatched roofs and no chimneys. It is not easy to keep clean when living in such a house and sleeping on the floor. Screens are lacking to keep out insects so that these people are often covered with insect bites. We have but to cross the Rio Grande into Mexico, our "good neighbor" to the south of us, to find many Indian tribes living in just this manner. The infant death rate among these Indians is said to be very high.

But a small part of the human family in the earth today has enough to eat. Many of China's and India's teeming millions die each year due to famine. In many other parts of the world, near-famine conditions prevail as a more or less constant state. The "struggle for existence" among the people of these places is a severe one. Contrary to popular propaganda, there exists in parts of Africa untouched by white settlement, or any white influence at all, poverty every whit as abject as that arising out of landlessness in South Africa. The utter poverty and prolonged physical deficiency of some of these people has had a far-reaching deteriorating effect upon both the bodies and the minds of the people.

The infant death rate is high in most of the world. A look at India will serve. Babies born in that overcrowded and hungry country have but little better than a one-to-four chance of surviving their first year of life. In some parts of the world the chances of surviving the first year of life are less than in India. If a baby survives its first year of life in India, it still has but a fifty-fifty chance of growing to maturity. In China, conditions are even worse.

In both of these overcrowded countries, there is not only food scarcity but there is a great lack of sanitation and in great portions of the population a neglect of the rudiments of personal hygiene. They are but little advanced, in these particulars, over Europe of the Middle Ages, and for somewhat the same reason—the stultifying effects of the theological dogma of the worthlessness of terrestrial life.

As humiliating as it may seem, it must be admitted that we, as a nation, are *below par* in every respect, and that our standards are empty of all value except for measuring varying degrees of ill-health.

Nothing has become more clear during the past twenty-five years than the fact that we are a nation of invalids and semi-invalids.

Examinations of school children and pre-school children show these all to be defective in one way or another and this by standards, which, as stated above, are of value only in measuring various degrees of ill-health. Examinations of young men for the army in 1917-18 and the examinations of the young men of today both by army examiners and the examiners for the N.Y.A., show that the defective school children of twelve and fifteen years ago, those of them who have reached maturity, are still defective. They have not "out-grown" their defects.

What of the young women? Are they in any better condition? Have they "out-grown" the defects they possessed as school children and pre-school children? Examinations of young women in the N.Y.A. reveal that they, too, are a bunch of scraps. They are largely unfit for any of the duties of life, whether in peace or in war.

Rejections from the army do not fully reveal the universal degeneracy in which we are immersed; for among those who are accepted as fit, the defects are only a little less marked. The army standard is a standard of disease, not of health. The flat chests, pimply faces, round shoulders, eye-glasses, plugged teeth, skinny, undeveloped bodies, and other signs of deterioration one sees among the conscripts, as well as in the regular army, point unmistakably to the fact that the army is made up of young men who are beginning to fall apart.

What is the meaning of the discharge from service in the last War of men over twenty-eight years old? It means that even those adjudged "fit" were so far down the scale of degeneracy that they could not stand up under the pseudo-training that the boys were given. As a nation we are physiologically botched and are becoming more so.

Mankind, every race and every sub-race of man, is capable of so much, yet we fall so far below those great capabilities because we do not have the means of turning out superior men and women and because we neglect the means that are at our disposal. Let us, in this country, not boast of our great advancement, for we have dedicated all of our channels of public information to the sacred task of keeping the people as a whole as grossly misinformed as the "smooth" operation of our profit system can tolerate. Ignorance and misinformation are everywhere, hence the poor nutrition of the great mass of Americans, despite a super-abundance of food all the year through.

If, in a few particulars, the life of the savage has advantages over that of the life of civilized man, in many particulars it is certainly inferior. There can be no doubt that the foods eaten by many savage and backward peoples are superior to those eaten by civilized man, but the scarcity of food among these people and the intensity of the struggle for existence among them often more than offset this simple advantage. Civilization is a mad house that sacrifices men, women and children upon the altars of commercialism—the overweaning desire for profits and more profits being the greatest motivating force in our capitalistic economy—but we do not advocate a return to savagery. Rather, would we revolutionize our civilization. Man is the center of the universe and we should build all of our institutions around him, around his needs and his highest interests, rather than build them, as now, around the *special interests* of the few who own the earth and exploit the many.

The greatest obstacle to living reform in the earth today, the greatest foe of dietary reform is not ignorance, of which there is much, but the desire of those who profit from the present evil practices and the means of carrying them on, to continue to reap rich financial harvests from pandering to the many harmful practices of the present conventional way of life. We are in serious need of economic and agricultural revolutions. Basic changes are required before we can hope to give every one the materials for a better and healthier life and before we can hope to reach them with the information that they need in order to make use of those materials. So long as our channels of public information and our educational system are in the hands of the, at present, economic royalists, so long as they conceive it to be their duty to serve the special interests of these private owners of the earth, rather than to serve the interests of the people as a whole, the truth about health, disease and healing will make slow progress in reaching the people.

In the meantime, we must make the best of what we have and not adopt a defeatist attitude. We must not throw up our hands and exclaim: "What's the use". The old copy-book maxim, "Rome was not built in a day," should be always in our minds and we should go on working for the ultimate attainment of our goal—*health for everybody*. Whatever stands in the way of the true advancement of man must give way to that which assists in his forward progress. Man, not the institutions, is sacred.

Amid the growing complexities of modern life, increasing numbers of bewildered people are searching for a more normal way of life. Perplexed, harrassed, even, in many instances, lost in the increasing chaos and confusion, they search more or less blindly and without definite direction for an illusive something that will lead them into a life of health, strength and happiness. A few are finding what they are searching for, but alas! all too many of them are shunted into blind alleys from which they never emerge, while many others fall by the way side.

The world is filled almost to overflowing with remedies for the miseries of mankind, there are panaceas galore, but they one and all prove disappointing when put to the test. ·The dogma that "man is what he eats," and the slogan, "diet does it," have misled and are misleading many. It seems to be very easy to convince great numbers of people that if they will but follow a particular scheme of diet or if they will eat certain almost magical articles of diet, they will grow into health and strength and maintain these to a very advanced period of life.

The so-called nutritionists are not, however, without competitors. The physical culturists are on hand with their many and varied systems of physical exercise, each of which is guaranteed to give you the health, strength, vigor and length of life you so much desire. The psychologists and psychiatrists have their own plans of salvation for a disease-ridden world. Indeed, we might enumerate these panaceas until we grow tired without exhausting the list.

The careful student of living and the careful observer of the results of the application of all these measures cannot but be struck by the fact that each and all of them are failures. This is not to say that they possess no value. It is not to assert that nobody derives any good from them. It is merely to say that all of this specialization and fragmentation fails to meet the needs of the problems that confront the modern man and woman. Something more is needed than diet, or than exercise, or than emotional adjustment. Life is very complex and no simple and single-factor formula for living can ever meet its many-sided requirements.

What is needed is a more comprehensive treatment of the whole problem of living in terms of a valid standard. A synthesis of inter-related and correlated living factors is required to provide the needs of the man, woman and child who is trying to find his way amid the complexities of our chaotic civilization. A vital need is a pattern of living normal for human beings that will cover the total needs of man and not merely one or two of his requirements. Only by taking into consideration all of the major factors of living and showing mankind how these may be related to his daily living, can we hope to enable him to solve the problems that confront him daily.

Not until we have learned to fully recognize the fact that all of the factors of living are interdependent and co-equal partners in a vital reciprocity can we expect to have superior nutrition and the superior health that grows out of this. As will be shown later, food is not nutrition. The purpose of the present book is not only to teach its readers much needed truths about food and feeding, but vital facts about other and related factors of nutrition. For, food alone, no matter how good, can never be made to constitute a complete answer to our nutritive needs.

The system of *Natural Hygiene* alone, of all the systems offered to the peoples of the earth as a solution for their problems of health, disease and healing, represents a synthesis of all the factor-elements of a normal life, hence, it alone can be relied upon to provide mankind with genuine salvation from its present deplorable state of ill-health and degeneracy. It is no single-method approach to the problems of life, but encompasses all of the basic needs of life.

The principles and the practices of *Natural Hygiene* are founded in the truths of physiology and biology and are sustained and perfected by all the valuable discoveries which mark their modern development. It is the function of *Natural Hygiene* to respect the laws of life and to defer to the inherent powers of the living organism. Any plan of living, in either health or disease, that is not based on the laws of life is destined to disappoint all who try it. Not until the minds of the people as a whole are fully awakened to a complete realization of the vital importance of the laws which govern the preservation and restoration of health of mind and body can we expect a cessation of the present reign of misery.

As natural laws admit of no exceptions, the subject of the laws of life, as these relate to our daily living and the health or disease that result therefrom, should be of the deepest interest to everyone. As upon obedience to the laws of life, or ignorant and wilful disregard of them, depend the happiness or misery of all mankind, we cannot afford to remain in ignorance of them. Prosperity may shower its brightest gifts on a man; wealth and art may combine to beautify and embelish his home; science and good literature may elevate his understanding and refine his tastes; the good and the wise may court his society; he may be exalted to the highest position to which his countrymen can elevate him, but of what avail are all of these advantages, if his body is weakly and wracked with pain and his home a scene of corroding anxiety and humiliating mortification caused by feeble, sickly, or defective children? Health, next to life, is man's most precious possession and without it his life is not likely to amount to much.

What is falsely called *"modern Scientific Medicine"* contents itself with experimental toying with a never ending succession of drugs and with symptoms, while utterly neglecting the laws of life. If the medical man ever thinks of hygiene at all it is as a "feeble auxiliary" to his poisons. He plies his victims with innumerable expedients of *medication,* suppressing symptoms and ignoring causes until the condition of the poor sufferer becomes so intolerable that even his most potent poisons will no longer afford the so much coveted temporary respite from misery. During the past twenty years the medical profession and the drug manufacturers have entertained us with a rapid succession of "wonder drugs," each of which enjoyed its brief heyday of popularity and then passed into that ever expanding Limbo reserved for the "cures" that pass in the night. Although they have held out to man great hope for the final eradication of suffering, the miracle drugs have proved to be as illusory as the drugs of yesteryear. There is no hope for man in poisons—violations of the laws of life cannot be remedied by poisons.

The purpose of this book is to point the people away from poisons to the normal things of life. The true Hygienist knows that the body needs and can use hygienic agents and influences and needs and can use no other. This is as true in disease as in health. If I succeed in convincing my readers that only those materials and influences that have a normal relation to life can be of constructive use to them in either health or disease; if I can make them realize that implicit obedience to the laws of life is their only salvation, that the results of one violation of the laws of life are not remedied by another violation of the same laws; if I can lead them to see that superior nutrition, which is the means of achieving and maintaining vigorous health, can be had only on nature's own terms and not by following some abnormal scheme concocted by some manufacturing house, or a group of commercially motivated salesmen; if I can point the way to better health for the children of this land, then, I will have accomplished my purpose in writing this book.

I have spent more than thirty two years in the exercise of my profession. For more than twenty-two years of this time I have conducted my own institution—Dr. Shelton's Health School—here in San Antonio, Texas. I have had a wide and varied experience in caring for both the well and the sick, the young and the old, the strong and the weak, the wise and the ignorant, the rich and the poor. As people have come to the Health School for care from many parts of the world, I have had experience that many others have lacked. I began my studies more than eleven years before I began my practice. I have spent well over forty years in intensive study of the subject of human nutrition. If great length of time spent in study and in applying the knowledge thus gained to the care of patients, entitle a man to speak with any degree of authority upon the subjects treated in this book, then, what I have to say is worthy of your careful attention and profound consideration. My great success in piloting my patients, including a great army of so-called "incurables" back to good health, is living evidence of the validity of the principles and practices herein set forth.

But I ask no reader to take anything in this book as truth merely because I have put it into the book. I ask, instead, that my readers think, investigate and test and find out for themselves whether what I say is true of false. Take no man as your guide. Truth alone should guide you. If I speak not the truth, if I err, if I am wrong, cast aside what I say and seek elsewhere. Mistake not authority for truth, but make truth your authority. Use your own thinking power and exercise your own ability to test all things and hold fast that which is good.

The Nutritional Basis of Life

CHAPTER I

Several generations of study of cell development and heredity have ignored almost completely the more important study of nutritional habits as these determine and pre-determine cell developments and affect reproduction and survival. The role of nutrition in integration, re-integration, and dis-integration has been shamefully neglected. For the most part, it has been taken for granted that it matters not what kind of food an organism consumes, so long as it consumes "enough" and more than "enough." Plenty of food and lack of food are chiefly considered as of importance. This places the most importance upon quantity rather than quality and kind.

Only recently have we begun to seriously investigate the physiological basis of life and the incidences of nutrition as they affect growth and reproduction, both in a physiological and pathological sense. It is true that hints of the role of nutrition in *health and disease* have come to thinking members of our race during the past several thousand years; but scientists have considered such things beneath their dignity.

Food supplies and food getting determine organisms in certain well defined directions. Different modes of nutrition are actually responsible for different modes of propagation. The end of nutrition is not merely to produce growth, but to satisfy those primordially indicated requisites of stability and normal function.

Life is dependent upon organization and organization is a product of growth or nutrition. It is through nutrition that we came into existence; through nutrition that we have whatever vigor we possess, and our health corresponds precisely to the quality of our nutrition. This is true of all plant and animal life. Living organisms, wherever found, with all their wonderful capacities and enjoyments, are merely the results of nutrition.

With perfect nutrition we have perfect organs, perfect functions and normal health; because the one is dependent upon and grows out of the other. This leads to the principle that: *the appropriate way to recover strength and vigor, is the same as we originally obtained these, through growth.* *We recover strength and vigor in the same way that we keep well, in the same way that the child grows into vigor and manhood. The power and processes that brought us into being, that sustain us in existence, that have caused us to grow through all the phases of life to manhood and womanhood, must restore us if anything does.*

What constitutes nutrition? Certainly the common thought that food and nutrition are the same thing is a fallacy that needs to be discarded. It is one thing to eat an abundance of good food, it is quite another thing to have good nutrition. Everyday we see examples of the fact that it is one thing to be able to eat an abundance of good food, but quite another to gain strength from the food. Food is one of the materials with which the processes of nutrition are carried on. Water is another and air is another. But neither one of these, nor all of them combined, constitutes nutrition.

Nutrition is a vital process carried on only by a living organism. It is a process of growth, development and invigoration. To eat good food and enough of it, to drink pure water and breathe pure air, in and of themselves are very desirable, but something more is needed in order to acquire health, strength and vigor.

Nutrition is function and we can have better nutritive function only when we have the capacity for better nutrition. Capacity cannot be bought. There are no drugs in the drug stores that can increase capacity, nor can they carry on the functions of life for us. The power to live, to breathe, to eat, to function resides within and not without us.

Food is of value only in its physiological connections with air, water, sunshine, rest and sleep, exercise or activity, cleanliness and wholesome mental and moral influences—in short, all the natural or normal circumstances which we know to be necessary for the preservation of health. Of these combined means contributing severely to the needs of the body, and each essential to it, it is enough to state that it would be impossible to assign to any over the rest a superior value, the simple fact being that each is indispensable and it is only in their plenary combination and harmonious co-adaptation to the wants of the body that real health is maintained or regained, once it has been lost. They constitute not only the only means that the powers of life can make use of in the preservation of health, but, also all that they can use in restoring health. They are nature's only remedial means.

Food is inert substance and, therefore, has no power to make living organisms. It cannot act, but is acted upon. The living organism uses what it can of the food consumed and rejects the rest. A particular food may be good, but to feed more of it than can be utilized, or more than is needed, on the theory that it builds this or that structure, or assists in the performance of this or that function, is worse than useless. The stuffing programs that are in vogue are wasteful of life—some of these consist of stuffing on all foods, others of stuffing on juices, or on foods rich in iron, or calcium, or vitamins, etc.

Almost daily we see skinny people eating abundantly of fattening foods without gaining an ounce; we see invalids eating freely of vitamin-rich foods and deriving no good therefrom. We see anemic patients eating iron without growing better; others eating large quantities of calcium-rich foods without making use of the calcium. *To eat it not always to appropriate.*

When it is discovered that the patient is not deriving the expected benefit from his abundance of vitamin-rich foods, recourse is had to vitamin extracts administered orally and to synthetic vitamins administered hypodermically or intravenously. When these fail, as they do, other tricks are tried. But the tricks do not enable the patient to utilize the vitamins. The assimilation and use of vitamins is a function of life and there is nothing outside of man that can do this for him. The *Hygienic* procedure is to first restore the man to a condition in which he is able to make full use of vitamins.

Physicians, friends and patient all agree that the latter is suffering for want of food, that he must be fed rich foods to build him up. Men who claim to understand the laws of organization and to be well versed in physiology feed such patients beef-steak, beef-tea, rich food, cod liver oil, etc., to "build them up." Everywhere the idea seems to prevail that food is nutrition, so that more food is urged.

If he does not gain weight and strength on his stuffing regimen, tonics and stimulants are added to the program. As these cannot add to his digestive and assimilative powers, but must inevitably lessen these, if their use is persisted in, the thin and weak invalid remains thin and weak, or grows thinner and weaker. The more he is stimulated, the weaker he grows. Nothing from without can add to man's nutritive capacities. Just as a large pile of lumber does not increase the productive capacity of the carpenter, so a large supply of food does not increase the digestive and assimilative capacity of the invalid. Before the desired results can be obtained, the capacities of the patient must be increased.

Capacity can be increased only by a wise use and economical expenditure of the forces of the organism. Power must be conserved if it is to be increased. Waste, friction, foolish expenditure must not be indulged. No doubt potential capacity is a matter of heredity, but the person whose capacity has been crippled or lowered can regain it only through the regular and normal processes of recuperation. Forcing measures and wasteful processes will not give added capacity.

Health is regained by precisely those primordial processes which originaly maintain it and these are referable solely to the inherent powers of the living organism. Health is directly dependent on the primary act of organization, that of constructing or building up, from elemental materials of the blood, the organs by which function is performed. If we are wise, we will consult nature's method of doing things and take into full account her materials and means of achieving her ends. It is presumptuous to do otherwise. If we would help, we must build as nature builds; if we would eliminate, we must do it as nature does it. As an indispensable basis, therefore, of the work of the *Hygienist*, we must endeavor to secure to the individual the full benefits of all the hygienic means, in their entire plenitude, for only thus can any health worthy the name be attained and/or maintained.

The nation is filled with patients who have tried many different diets and many different feeding programs and have failed to derive benefit therefrom. They have tried the vitamin preparations, mineral concentrates, special articles of diet, various so-called "aids to digestion," etc., all to no avail. They have stuffed themselves on all foods, they have over-eaten on particular foods, they have used special food preparations, they have given the principle that "man is what he eats" a thorough test, and it has been found wanting. Has not the time arrived when we should begin to devote more attention to the processes by which man appropriates his food and cease concentrating our whole attention upon the food eaten? Before we feed a man, let us be certain that he can appropriate what we feed him. What is to be gained by merely passing food through the man without having it digested and assimilated?

To feed a man the theoretically necessary number of calories each day is not to guarantee that he shall derive the calories from his food. If the food ferments in his digestive tract, he will derive no calories from it. To eat abundantly of high-grade protein and have it putrefy in the digestive tract is not to derive the required amino acids therefrom. If we feed the man according to theoretical needs and not according to actual capacity (*As he is, so shall he eat*) we do him great injury. Do we not daily see chronic invalids stuffing themselves on "plenty of good nourishing food" to build up their strength, only to see them grow progressively weaker? Is it not a common experience in *Hygienic* institutions and in *Hygienic* practice, to see invalids gain strength on less food?

Instead of studying nature and her laws with the idea of using her laws, conditions and materials constructively, we seem to study her in an effort to discover how to cheat her. Like the business man who told his lawyer, "I do not want to know how to obey the law, but how I may safely break it," we seek not to obey the laws of life, but to disobey them. Often it is as important to know what not to do as to know what to do. Thousands of patients are killed yearly and many thousands more are irreparably injured because their physicians do not know what *not to do*. As the practitioners of all schools of so-called healing are wedded to the dogma that "it is right to do evil that good may result," they are forever engaged in doing the wrong things. Their patients must suffer accordingly.

There are times when one should not eat, there are conditions under which no food should be taken. It is as important to know when to abstain from food as it is to know when to eat and how much. Primordially, eating serves to secure to the body the requisite elements of nutrition and there is nothing to be gained by eating when no food is required, or when food cannot be digested and assimilated. Abstinence from food (fasting) is one of the most common occurrences in nature and is resorted to under a varied number of conditions and circumstances.

Life is More Than Food

CHAPTER II

A system is made up of principles of action quite as much as of materials of use. Principles are the bases of action and false principles are fecund with evil. One false principle can disjoint a whole system. Indeed, one false principle, entering into a system, can produce more mischief than a thousand so-called "false facts." A false principle can confuse and bewilder and render mysterious the truth until every conceivable absurdity is accepted, believed and acted upon. A system that is devoid of correct principles of action, one that operates from erroneous principles, must, of necessity, always act wrongly. Its actions must be in harmony with its principles.

The differences between the uses of diet, exercise, sunshine, water, rest, sleep, temperature, mental factors, etc., by the *Hygienic* school and their uses by other schools of thought, are determined by the respective principles of application of the various schools. Everybody eats, but everybody is not, thereby, a Hygienist. Breathing by everybody does not constitute everybody *Hygienists*. For example, *Hygienists* work upon the principle that "as a man is, so shall he eat," whereas, the dietitians and the various schools of so-called healing that make any use of diet, assert that "man is what he eats."

The late Dr. Henry Lindlahr is credited with having first declared that "man is what he eats," but the dogma is much older than Dr. Lindlahr, as is easily shown. In an editorial in *Life Illustrated* for April 25, 1875, Dr. Trall quotes the following words from some unidentified source: "As a man eateth so is he." This is the way the dogma that "man is what he eats" was expressed during the last century. Early in this century Dr. E. M. Woolsey wrote in *Self-Help* (York, Pa.) under the title, "Man is What He Eats." As he quotes this dogma, it is reasonable to suppose that he borrowed it from some other source. He says, *"Man is what he eats.* Morality, national and individual, is but a question of diet."

An echo of this dogma comes to us regularly over the air on the grape-nuts flakes program, when "California" Carlson drones to the children: "If you wanna be like Hoppy, you gotta eat like Hoppy." This is just another way of saying: "Man is what he eats."

Hygienists repudiate this whole idea and set up, instead, the rule, as expressed by Dr. Robert Walter, that "as a man is, so shall he eat." Graham expressed this same principle in his rule that the weakest organ of the body should be made the standard by which to feed the patient or the so-called well person. Trall expressed the same principle when he laid down the rule of practice, not only that the feeding of patients, but all other care of them, should be in keeping with the capacities and needs of the body under the conditions as these exist at the time. What was to be fed or supplied to the body was to be modified according to the conditions.

At no time should anyone, and still less should patients be fed according to any arbitrary standard, such as the assumed need for so many calories a day, or the need for a certain amount of protein a day, or the asserted need for certain minimum requirement of this or that vitamin each day. Due regard for the capacities and abilities of the patient to make use of the food eaten must always be had. Just what is gained by feeding a patient the theoretically required number of calories, for example, when he is unable to digest and assimilate any of them, is something that has not yet been explained.

Food is to be used to supply the nutritive needs of the body, and what it needs is determined by its constitution, its current condition and by the work it performs. To assume, as has long been done, that "food makes the man," and hence, "the character of the man," and to feed according to this absurdity is not to achieve desirable results.

The differences between these two principles of application are precisely the differences between making the coat for the man and making the man for the coat; between hewing the foot to the boot, and making the boot to fit the foot. In *Hygienic* practice we insist that the materials of life shall be subordinated to the living organism and not the living organism subordinated to the materials.

Man is of more consequence than the matter around him; life is more than food and the body more than raiment. It follows from this that a knowledge of the man is of more consequence than a knowledge of anything around him. Man is the active force of nature, and his future is wrapped up in his doings. The elements of success or of failure are in the man. The *potentials* in the acorn and not the soil in which it grows, give us an oak tree. No possible manipulation of the soil, or of sun and water, can cause a millet seed to produce an oak tree.

Food does not make the man. Fish do not make brains, as was formerly held. Beans do not make muscles. If these things were true, then unlimited brain and muscle could be made, for both fish and beans are abundant. Eating squash will not produce a soft head, and eating liver will not produce giant livers. Food is only material for use by the man in building himself, just as lumber is material for use by the workers in building a house.

If a man is born stupid, all the fish in the ocean will not make him otherwise. To advocate the use of this or that or the other food on the ground that will give strength, feed particular organs, or develop peculiar characteristics, is to advocate and practice fallacy. To employ foods from this standpoint is unhygienic and unscientific, and will end in disappointment.

Muscles are built by the body in response to exercise, not by stuffing on muscle-building foods. No Hercules ever developed from herculean eating. He developed out of herculean exercise. Not every man is a potential Hercules. No doubt muscular potential is largely a matter of heredity, but no man ever realized his full potentiality without exercise. That exercise without food will not build muscle goes without saying, but the process is still vital and neither of these factors do the actual building of muscle.

The laboratory man can easily demonstrate that molasses and butter, sugar and fat make heat, and yet the cold and bloodless one eats these in abundance and daily grows colder. This and like absurdities grow out of the fallacy that "It is the food that makes the man, and hence the character of the man will be immediately changed by a change of food." This fundamental fallacy underlies the dietary notions of most of the schools of healing and of all of the dietetic schools.

It is not what one eats that invigorates one, but what one digests and appropriates; hence, to know how to improve digestion and assimilation is of more importance than to know what foods to feed. Air, food and water constitute the materials out of which living organisms are made and, although the quality of the material is very important, it is not more important than the process of using it. Good digestion is as necessary as good food, and good assimilation is equally important.

By the foregoing it is not intended to convey the thought that food is not important, nor that it is not a vitally important determining factor in health and disease, in development and growth, and in the kind of organism we produce. It is merely intended to emphasize that food, important as it is, is but one of several needs of life and that it is subordinate to life. Man uses food—food does not use man. It is, therefore, essential that we do not lose sight of the importance of the man who is eating the food and that we do not concentrate all of our attention upon the food that is eaten.

Foodstuffs

CHAPTER III

Foodstuffs, as we eat them, are composed of a few complex substances which are classified as proteins, carbohydrates, fats, organic salts, vitamins, water, and indigestible portions, or waste, to which the terms bulk or roughage are commonly applied. To be a true food, the substance eaten must not contain harmful ingredients. The leaf of the tobacco plant contains all of these food elements, but, in addition to these, it contains nicotine, one of the most virulent poisons known to man, and several other poisons; hence, tobacco is not a true food. To eat a large salad of tobacco leaves, as we do of lettuce leaves, would be to become very ill and, if we were not killed outright, life would, at least, be seriously endangered.

The term protein is derived from *Proteus* (I take the first rank), and protein substance was so named because it was regarded as the commencement and starting point of all animal tissues. Out of this original conception of the importance of protein, whether true or not, grew many mistakes that were corrected in time, but which tend to arise again from time to time, to harrass the seeker after dietary truth. Contrary to current popular teaching, bull-beef and boar-steak are not the only sources of protein. Indeed, animal tissues are not the best sources of proteins, as we shall see later on. There is so much fallacy afloat about proteins that it will be necessary to consider this substance in greater detail in subsequent chapters.

The carbohydrates are starches and sugars, of which the body can use only sugar. When starches are eaten, these must first be converted into sugar in the process of digestion, before they are useful to the body. Sugar does not mean commercial extractives of the beet, cane, milk, maple tree, etc., nor yet does it mean syrup, which is the boiled and condensed sap of the tree or cane, nor honey. While all of these substances are sugar, they are not ideal forms of sugar for our use. Dates, figs, prunes, sweet grapes, sweet apples, persimmons, well ripened bananas, raisins, etc., are the ideal sources from which to secure the body's sugar requirements. Cereals,

legumes, tubers, etc., are sources of starch. Nuts contain carbohydrate either in the form of sugar or in the form of starch. Theoretically, carbohydrates are burned in the body to supply heat and
energy.

The common practice of taking almost nothing but denatured
carbohydrates—white flour and white flour products, white rice,
white sugar, demineralized corn meal, etc.—guarantees that the average American is subsisting on a diet that has been robbed of much
of its normal mineral content and most of its vitamins. Indeed, in
some of these foods no minerals or vitamins are left. For optimum
nutrition, our carbohydrates should be natural—that is they should
not be denatured.

Although the body can manufacture most of its fats out of carbohydrates and proteins, it seems that certain fatty acids may be necessary for optimum nutrition which the body seems unable to make
for itself. For this reason, fats are important in the diet. Butter,
cream, lard, and related animal fats are the most commonly used
fats in this country. Oleomargarine is rapidly supplanting butter in
the diets of Americans, primarily because during World War II, the
dairy industry and the government went crazy and ran the price of
butter up to prohibitive levels where it has since remained. Many
vegetarians have turned from the use of butter (an animal fat) to
the use of oleomargarine (a vegetable fat). Oleomargarine is a refined fat, comparable to lard and cooking compounds, which is "re-
inforced" with synthetic vitamins. It is far from being a wholesome
article of diet and the vegetarian will do well to avoid it. Oleomargarine will not keep without the addition of a preservative and
this renders it further unfit for food.

The oils of nuts and of the avocado are eaten with these foods
and constitute choice sources of easily digested emulsified oils. If
nuts are eaten abundantly, there is no need to add oil from any other
source to the diet, as these will easily supply the body with all the
fat required. If other oils are desired, the following vegetable oils
are tasty and full of food value and may be used by the vegetarian,
who does not want to use butter or cream; olive oil, peanut oil,
soybean oil, sunflower seed oil, sesame oil, corn oil and cotton-
seed oil. Only cold pressed or virgin olive oil or seed oils should be
used. Refined oils, having been deprived of their minerals and

vitamins, and having been impaired in the process of refining, should be avoided.

The minerals—calcium (lime), phosphorus, sulphur, magnesium, manganese, iodine, copper, iron, sodium, silicon, chlorine, flourine, nickle, etc.—serve a number of important purposes in the body. Besides entering into the constitution of the various tissues of the body, as calcium and phosphorus in the bones and teeth, and iron in the blood, and being important ingredients in the various secretions of the body, as chlorine in the gastric juice and iodine in thyroxin, they assist in maintaining normal osmotic pressure within the body, are used in carrying oxygen (copper and iron) and aid in the excretion of waste from the body. They also assist in maintaining the normal alkalinity of the blood.

Some of these minerals, like copper and nickle, are present in the body and in foodstuffs as mere traces and are called "trace minerals." Their importance is out of all proportion to the amount present in foods or in the body. Certain of the endocrine secretions are useless without the presence of one or more of these trace minerals.

The richest sources of minerals are green vegetables, fruits and nuts. Certain animal foods, like eggs and milk are abundant in them, but the milk supplied today is practically all pasteurized and this has much of its mineral content ruined for use. The method of forcing egg production now in use (a chicken feed company states that the hen is "nothing but an egg factory") assures the egg-eating portions of our public very inferior eggs, that are deficient both in minerals and vitamins. Grains are commonly well supplied with certain of the minerals. Many vegetables in common use contain twice as much calcium as milk and, if eaten raw, instead of being cooked ("pasteurized") supply their calcium in available form.

Vitamins, of which there are several, are not foods, but accessory food substances that are used by the body in its work of assimilating or using foods. In their absence, the body either makes no use of the food elements at all or else makes a very faulty use of them. This means a retardation of growth, faulty or distorted growth, poor structure, deterioration of structure already built, failing function and the so-called "deficiency diseases."

Our best sources of vitamins are green and yellow vegetables and vegetables that are white and red and purple, and fruits and nuts.

To guarantee that the vitamins are obtained unimpaired these foods should be eaten uncooked and without being processed. Vitamins are very unstable substances and are easily destroyed.

The cataylzers—enzymes, hormones, vitamins—though present in minute amounts, are substances which are capable of inducing wonderful and most important effects upon organic matter. Indeed, these substances seem to contain the most indispensable guiding principles influencing organic form. The hydrochloric acid-pepsin of the stomach are capable of changing quantities of albumen into colloidal solutions, thus fitting them for further elaboration by the organism. Enzymes have been termed the tools of the cells. Their number is legion, but chemistry cannot produce them. They are found only as the products of protoplasm of living cells and are known chiefly by their relations. They are always found in association with proteins, but mineral salts seem to be essential to their usefulness. Enzymes appearing originally, as by-products of photosynthetic and associated metabolic processes of the plant, are highly complex and delicately poised substances. Hormones are manufactured by the endocrine glands out of substances contained in the blood, but they must first be contained in the food. This means that the vital potencies of these internal secretions are derived from plants, which alone possess the necessary synthetic powers of manufacture.

Chlorophyll, which is probably never formed by the animal body (green blooded animals derive their chlorophyll from plants the same as do red-blooded animals), is very extensively taken in with vegetable foods, and forms the basis from which a large number of animal pigments, including the widely distributed pigment, hemoglobin (the red coloring matter of the blood), are built up. Since chlorophyll is the source of our respiratory pigment, especially of the vital hemoglobin, all efforts to substitute animal protein for chlorophyll (as is frequently done in anemia) must always result in difficulties. The normal source of chlorophyll is green plants, eaten as foods. Commercial products—extracted chlorophyll and synthetic chlorophyll—that are on the market, are expensive, inferior, and unnecessary. It is not likely that chlorophyll can be extracted from plants by complex chemical and other processes without serious damage to it. Even in anemia, the green plant, especially in the raw state, is superior to commercial products.

Organic Vs. Inorganic

CHAPTER IV

"Suum cuique tributio,"—Give to each its own. The body requires for the nourishment of its tissues, substances which are identical with them in essence. But even this is not enough so far as the animal body is concerned. For the animal, substances are food or not, less from their ultimate essence than from their proximate forms. The same essential elements that constitute the human body are to be found in the soil and in water and air, but the elements of the soil do not constitute food for man. It is first necessary that these elements be elaborated into certain organic compounds by the transforming power of the plant before they can be used by the animal organism. The compounds made by the chemist differ in their internal structure and in the relative positions of their component molecules from those elaborated by the plant and are worthless as food for man and beast.

The direct transformation of inorganic matter into living animal tissue is impossible. There must always occur the intermediate phenomenon of plant life. Vegetables alone can transform the inorganic chemicals of the air and soil into living structure, so that the animal is forced to feed upon the plant or upon another animal that has fed upon the plant. Water and the oxygen of the air are the only exceptions to this fact. The vegetable is intermediate between the minerals and animals. Let us look at this more in detail.

Soil is full of minerals, the same minerals that are required by the body in building its own structure and in carrying on its functions. But you cannot supply your mineral requirements by eating a handful of soil each day. The air is full of nitrogen and carbon, but you cannot take these from the air and synthesize them into proteins, carbohydrates and fats. Nor, can you take these elements of soil, air and water and manufacture vitamins of them. The work of manufacturing amino acids from nitrogen belongs exclusively to the plant. The work of manufacturing starches and sugars from the carbon contained in the air is also the office of the plant. The plant alone can take the minerals of the soil and turn out organic salts. The plant alone can manufacture vitamins.

We cannot manufacture foods in the laboratory. Between biology and chemistry there is a great difference. We must recognize that biological growth and chemical synthesis are divided by an impassible gulf. The synthetically constructed "foodstuffs" of the laboratory are absolutely unfit for use. Nature's biological laboratory turns out her food products by processes that are unknown to the chemist. Biological synthesis and chemical synthesis are not identical processes and do not turn out identical products.

The plan of nature is first soil, then vegetables, then animals and man. When the laboratory men try to reverse this order and feed the soil to us without it first being incorporated into the vegetable and being prepared in suitable and acceptible compounds, it does not work well. It does seem that old Mother Nature will have to stay on the job for a long while yet.

First, we have stone, which disintegrates and forms soil; then we have vegetation, at first, represented only by the *pioneer plants*. These die and are returned to the soil, so that each generation of vegetables feeds the next. Finally, there appear vegetables that are capable of sustaining the higher animals. Here, then, is the order: rock, silt, primary vegetation, higher vegetation, animal. Valuable as are the elements of rock to the vegetable, you will derive very little comfort and satisfaction out of trying to raise vegetables on rock. First, it must be broken down and made into silt. Then, the work of the pioneer plants is essential. When we reflect upon the fact that it is not until after the "pioneer plants" have broken down the disintegrated rock and prepared the way, that the higher forms of vegetable life can exist in the soil, a fact the organic gardeners are emphasizing, we readily see the impossibility of feeding the human body on the chemist's products of the rock. You will not get much satisfaction out of attempting to raise animals and children on rock, no matter how finely ground.

Minerals, as these are supplied by the drug store, are never found in the human body. Lime, iron, sodium, copper, magnesium, phosphorous, iodine, etc., are normal constitutents of the human body but they can be appropriated and transformed into human tissue only when they are provided in the form of organic salts. Inorganic salts and "free" minerals are simply poisons. Indeed, some of these minerals in the "free" state, or in the form of inorganic salts, are virulent poisons. The poisonous character of phosphorous and iodine is well known.

The fact that so-called "over doses" of synthetic vitamins, or their use over a lengthy period of time occasions so-called toxic symptoms is undeniable evidence that they are non-usable substances. All summer long the cow, deer, horse, or other ruminant may eat grass and other green foods in enormous quantities and thus receive daily all the vitamins in heavy doses and develop no signs of toxic symptoms. Toxic symptoms flow from the use of the chemist's synthetic imitations of vitamins, just as they flow from the use of his imitations of the salts of the plant.

Among those who have not outgrown the *curing* delusion, there are many who believe that they can usurp nature's prerogatives and do her work for her. Among these are those who style themselves *biochemists. Bio-chemistry,* as the word implies, is the chemistry of life, or the chemistry of living organisms. This cult, originated many years ago by Schuessler of Germany, attempts to maintain or restore health by supplying the body with the materials lacking in the parts affected. As Schuessler, himself, said, "biochemistry endeavors to correct the physiological chemistry when it has deviated from the normal state." He also states, that, "anyone who will consider without prejudice the end to be attained, and the ways and means, will come to see that the biochemical remedies when used after proper selection, are sufficient for the cure of all diseases curable by internal remedies."

To do what the "biochemist" seeks to do, if it were possible for man to do it, would require a far greater knowledge of "physiological chemistry" than either Schuessler or anybody now living have. Schuessler put forth his theories at a time when far less was known of the chemistry of living organisms than is known today. His "remedies" were few and simple, when compared with the "remedies" of the present day "biochemist." But, he, like his successors, ignored the fact that the normal and only source of "natural materials" of the animal is the plant kingdom. Like Schuessler, the present-day "biochemist" goes to the chemical laboratory for his "remedies."

The so-called "biochemist" has a strong tendency to abandon, or ignore biochemistry and resort to just everyday chemistry (inorganic chemistry). Schuessler, the Homeopathist, who was the first "biochemist" started the world off on this false course when he put forth the theory that "the biochemical method supplies the curative efforts of nature with the natural materials lacking in the parts affected."

The "biochemist" looks upon practically all "diseases" as results of deficiencies and ignores the patent evidence that the symptoms of practically all of them are symptoms of poisoning. Even the deficiencies, where these do exist, are more often the results of poisoning, than lack of materials in the foods eaten. In such cases, it is not possible to supply deficiencies, except by first eliminating the poisoning.

While Schuessler confined himself to the use of "cell salts," that is, to the administration of minerals necessary to build and repair body structure, his successors have departed from his dictum that, the "biochemical remedies" he used, "when properly used," after "proper selection are sufficient for the cure of all disease curable by internal remedies," and make use of minerals of which he knew not, and of vitamins of which he never dreamed. They also employ amino acids and chlorophyll, the first of which was probably unknown to him. *Biochemistry* has become very complex since the Master passed away and the methods of treatment have become correspondingly complex, even if not more successful. The failures of "biochemical" treatment attest to its inadequacy to meet the requirements of the sick. Its successes, like those of Christian Science, and the regular program of drugging, are those of nature—we cannot usurp nature's prerogative of healing.

The building materials with which the body is built, maintained and repaired must be supplied by the food we eat. Schuessler and his devotees employed and do employ free minerals and inorganic salts, such as they could provide in the laboratory, rather than organic salts as these are provided in foods. In more simple English, "biochemistry," as Schuessler promulgated it, is a drugging system. It did not propose to supply deficiencies by feeding natural foods, but by dosing with non-usable minerals. Even now the "biochemists" are the backbone of the synthetic vitamin industry. Synthetic "vitamins" are drugs, not vitamins. They are non-usable, hence toxic.

It may be true, as Dr. Tilden wrote, that, Schuessler's salts do little harm, but it is certainly true, as he also wrote, that, "the harm it ("biochemistry") does is to entertain the minds of the doctor and his patient when they should be learning to think in the *language of correct living.*"

"Too many physicians are still moulding mud-pies in the kindergarten of their imaginations and delusions," says Tilden. The sick do not need *scientific hod-carriers* and *bricklayers.* There is a great gap between the calcium salts of the foods turned out by nature and the calcium salts of the laboratory and no chemist can bridge that gap. Altogether too many chemists are suffering from a self-destructive egomania. It is one thing to supply the body with iron in food and quite another to take iron compounds prepared in the chemical laboratory. We should go no further back than the plant kingdom, from which to secure the minerals with which to build and maintain the body—we should cease our efforts to reverse the established order of nature.

Amino Acids

CHAPTER V

When proteins are fully digested in the human digestive tract, the result is a group of simpler compounds which are acceptable to the blood and tissues of the body and which are known as amino acids. These are organic acids containing nitrogen. As these are substances of which all proteins, plant and animal, are synthesized, they are often called the "building stones" of the body. Many proteins are known, but all of them are made up of different combinations and varying proportions of the amino acids. Just as the many thousands of words in the English language are made up of various combinations of the twenty-six letters in the alphabet, so the many proteins are built up of various combinations of the amino acids.

The body cannot use protein as such. When proteins are split up into their constituent amino acids, the body may then use these amino acids as building stones with which to construct its own peculiar types of protein. Many different types of protein are taken as food, but none of them are human proteins. If absorbed directly into the blood as proteins, they would not be able to suply the protein needs of the body, but on the contrary, would constitute foreign materials and would occasion pathological *reactions,* such as are seen in *anaphylaxis* and *allergy.*

Twenty-seven or twenty-eight amino acids have been recovered from proteins, as follow: Glycine or Glycocoll, Alamine, Amino-butyric acid, Amino-valeric acid, Valine, Norleucine, Leucine, Isolucine, Serine, Threonine, Aspartic acid, Glutamic acid, Hydroxy-glutamic acid, Cystine, Methionine, Phenylalanine, Tyrosine, Di-iodo-tyrosine, Thyroxine, Lysine, Arginine, Ornithine, Citrulline, Tryptophane, Histadine, Proline, Hydroxyproline. Not all of these are found in any one protein; proteins being made up of varying combinations and proportions of several of them.

The proteins of animals and plants are constituted of the various amino acids in a specific pattern for each species with some slight differences between the proteins of the sexes within the species.

Not merely every species of animal and plant has its own specific protein, but also within each animal and plant each organ and part has its own peculiar protein or proteins. The amino acid content of the different tissues of the body differs as much as do the tissues. It has been estimated that there are a thousand six hundred different proteins in the human body. A similar protein complexity exists within the bodies of other animals, and within the bodies of plants. Each plant has several different parts—seeds, fruits, leaves, etc., each having their own specific protein. Many parts of plants and animals possess two or more proteins. All of this is to say that the protein in one organ or part of an animal or plant is not the same as the protein in another organ or part in the same plant or animal. Due to these differences, the proteins of the different parts of plants or animals do not all have the same nutritive value.

When proteins have been broken down into their constitutent amino acids by the processes of digestion, these are taken up by the blood stream and carried to all parts of the body, the cells of the body taking them from the blood stream as required in building protein—human proteins in the case of man. Each tissue appropriates the requisite amino acids in the required amounts and proportions to build protein peculiar to itself. Thus, the reader will see that proteins are not built out of proteins, but out of amino acids. The body cannot use proteins as such, but must first tear down the complex proteins of foodstuffs and make its own proteins. Nut protein, egg protein, cereal protein, milk protein, etc., are not human proteins. In order to build human proteins out of foreign proteins, these must be reduced to their "building stones" and these "stones" used in building up the new structures. Foreign proteins, if introduced into the bloodstream, without first undergoing the process of digestion, that is, without being reduced to amino acids, are rank poisons.

Amino acids are not interchangeable. Each one is specific in its function, so that one cannot be made to substitute for another. For example, no superabundance of the amino acid constitutents of proteins will compensate for deficiency of tyrosine and tryptophane, and such deficient proteins are unable to maintain the integrity of living tissues.

Some proteins will support normal growth, maintenance and reproduction. Such proteins are said to be *adequate* or *complete*. A protein that supports maintenance only is considered *partially adequate* or *partially complete*. A protein that will support neither growth nor maintenance is considered *inadequate* or *incomplete*. Thus, a protein is considered *adequate, partially adequate,* or *inadequate* depending on its ability to support growth, maintenance and reproduction. This is described as the "biological value" of the protein.

The method of testing the biological value of the various proteins is to separate and isolate them from the foods in which they naturally exist and feed them as the exclusive source of protein. For example, an animal may be fed on a diet that contains no protein except the lactalbumen of milk, or the diet may contain no protein save the glutenin of wheat. Thus the "biological value" of particular proteins is determined by feeding test.

A protein is said to have high physiologic or biologic value the smaller the amount of it required to supply the needs of the animal. Based upon this standard, whole egg is ranked as 94; milk, 85, liver and kidney, 77; heart, 74; muscle meat, 69; whole wheat 64; potato, 67; rolled oats, 65; whole corn, 60; white flour 52; navy beans, 38. By this standard, vegetable proteins in general are said to be nearly always inferior to those of animal origin. The proteins of peanuts and soy beans are listed as exceptions, their proteins being complete. There are no appreciable differences between the muscle meat of cow, hog or sheep. Notice that nuts, which certainly form an important part of man's normal diet, are ignored in this classification, while grains and legumes, which certainly form no part of his normal diet, are sharply contrasted with animal foods. Berg says that the protein of potatoes is more efficiently utilized by the body than that of flesh. Hinhede found potato protein to be of very high value. Others have confirmed his findings. Nuts and the green plants possess proteins of the highest value.

While the biologic value of a protein is determined by feeding tests, its value depends upon its amino acid content. Of the known amino acids, some ten or twelve are declared to be essential to human and animal life. These are called *essential* amino acids, because the body is unable to synthesize them. The other amino acids, called *non-essential,* the body is able to make for itself by reducing some of the more complex amino acids, providing, of course, that an excess of the essential ones is eaten. Elvehjern has shown that some of these so-called non-essential amino acids may be needed for optimum growth. Actually the classification of amino acids into *essential* and *non-essential* is misleading, as the body needs all of them and is unable to produce any of them out of raw materials.

Gelatin is a protein derived from certain parts of the animal. It is very inadequate. Animals fed on this protein exclusive of other sources of protein not only do not grow but are unable to maintain themselves and die. Zein, a protein of corn, is equally inadequate. Each of these proteins is lacking in certain essential amino acids. Both of them are useful to the animal body, but they require to be supplemented from other sources if life is to be maintained and growth occur.

This brings us to a fact of vital importance in this discussion: namely, *the deficiencies of one protein may be made good by another protein which possesses the amino acids lacking in the first.* Two proteins, each of which lacks the same amino acids will not complement each other, but two incomplete proteins, each of which possesses the amino acids lacking in the other will, together, constitute a complete protein. Unless the diet of a man or an animal is confined to one protein there is not likely to be a lack of any of the essential amino acids.

Zein is not the only protein in corn. Lactalbumen is not the only protein in milk. Almost every known source of protein contains two or more proteins. Milk and eggs each have two proteins. Wheat has several. Each nut possesses more than one protein. This brings us to a second fact that is of vital importance to this discussion: namely, *one protein in a food may fully complement another protein in the same food so that the two proteins, together, constitute a complete protein.* This is not so of the proteins of grains, nor of the proteins of a mixture of several grains. But it is true of grains plus an abundance of green vegetables. Green vegetables contain small amounts of the highest grade proteins and these supplement the deficiencies in many other foods. In the early spring, grazing animals derive practically their whole protein supply from green vegetables—grasses and weeds. In order to do this, they must consume these foods in great quantities, a thing for which man lacks the capacity. Man must, therefore, derive much of his protein supply from more concentrated sources. As man must have his daily supply of greenstuff, if he is to maintain good health, he can supplement his other proteins with proteins from this source. For example, if a man desires to live upon whole grains, he can do this only by eating large quantities of green vegetables with the grains. Experiments show that best results are obtained when the greens in the diet constitute more than fifty percent of the total food intake.

For experimental purposes, in determining the value of the different proteins, single isolated proteins are fed. In actual practice, neither man nor animal lives upon a single or isolated protein. They not only eat a variety of foods made up of a variety of proteins, but they eat foods, each of which contains two or more proteins. In regular practice we do not consume casein as our sole source of protein, nor do we live upon an exclusive grain diet. This brings us to a third vitally important fact in this discussion: namely, *we do not live upon one protein food, but upon the total protein content of our varied diet.* We do not have to ask ourselves: is this particular protein an adequate protein? nor; do the proteins contained in this particular protein-food collectively constitute an adequate protein? We need only ask: *Does the total protein content of the diet as a whole supply all the protein needs of my body?* If the *ensemble* of the protein intake is adequate, this is sufficient.

Animal experimenters are prone to overemphasize the importance of the substances they use with which to supplement inadequate diets and ignore, almost wholly, the natural order of feeding. Milk is a very handy item of food and is used very much in supplementing experimental diets. It usually suffices to render adequate the inadequate diets fed to the animals, hence the experimenters are prone to overemphasize the value and importance of milk and to ignore the obvious fact that, in nature animals secure adequate diets without resort to milk after they are weaned. Their experimental diets are almost never the diets of the people, nor are they the diets of animals in nature. The tendency of this class of experiments is to mislead. There are many other foods that may be used that will render adequate an inadequate diet.

In a certain series of experiments dogs were fed upon deficient diets. They failed to grow normally. To the diet of some of the dogs a quantity of milk was added. These dogs grew and developed normally. The dogs that received no milk were stunted and poorly developed. It would be folly to reason from this that dogs require milk for normal development, for we know that dogs can and do develop normally without getting any milk after they are weaned. All that such an experiment proves is that milk added to an otherwise deficient diet will render the diet adequate. But there are hundreds of other ways of rendering diets adequate as all animals in the wild state are aware. Indeed, it is possible and probable that many of the other means of rendering the diets adequate are superior to milk. Milk, after the normal suckling period has ended, is far from being an unmixed blessing.

Experiments with single, isolated proteins would easily lead the unwary to believe that the elephant, cow, horse, buffalo, bison, deer, rabbit, and other strictly vegetable eating animals can not live and grow on their vegetable diets, but actually we know that they do very well on such diets. This is because they never attempt to live on individual isolated proteins, but eat a varied diet, in which one protein corrects another.

The amino acid requirements of different animals doubtless differ very much, just as the amino acid requirements of an adult animal differ greatly from the amino acid requirements of the same animal when it is rapidly growing. When a protein has been shown to be adequate for a certain species of animal, this is all that has been shown. It cannot be said to be adequate or inadequate for another species until it has been tested on the other animal. When foods are tested on rats, the results of the tests are not fully applicable to man.

The proteins of bananas as are said to be very incomplete, yet there is a South American parrot that lives upon a monodiet composed exclusively of bananas and he lives to a very ripe old age. Banana proteins prove adequate for him. In the tropics convalescent patients, recovering from the wasting effects of typhoid or other fever, are often fed a banana diet and gain weight and strength rapidly. Banana proteins must be more adequate for man than the experiments with the rats indicate. Of course, neither the parrots nor the patients eat the isolated protein. They eat the banana.

The tendency, today, is to emphasize meat (flesh), eggs and milk as sources of proteins, and to disregard, or even, to discount all other sources of amino acids. Every effort is made to convince the people, who, by the way, seem to require but little convincing, that they are normally and constitutionally, carnivores, hence animal foods are their best foods.

The high biological value of egg, milk and flesh proteins is not to be denied. There are, however, other considerations, which need not be discussed at this place, for rejecting the carnivorous diet. I shall here consider only the assertions made for one of these animal foods as a source of amino acids.

Let us come to flesh foods. It is argued that flesh proteins contain all of the essential amino acids and are, therefore, superior to plant proteins, many of which are poor in some of the needed amino acids and over rich in others. It is also asserted that animal proteins are more easily digested and assimilated than plant proteins. Flesh, therefore, is overemphasized in many quarters as a food for man. Here again, the natural order of feeding is ignored. Is flesh a complete protein? Berg says: "this cannot be accepted as a positive fact as regards the protein of individual muscles, only as regards the aggregate proteins of the animal body used as food." Abderhalden also points out this fact. Berg says this is especially true if flesh is not accompanied with a large supply of base-forming foods. He points out that "carnivorous animals, living in a state of nature, secure a supply of bases by drinking the blood of their victims and devouring the bones and cartilages as well as the flesh." It is also true that wild carnivores consume considerable quantities of fruits, berries and buds. They especially eat such foods in the Autumn. Cats are often observed to eat vegetable foods and this is done, contrary to popular notions, while in health, not when sick.

It has long been known that if a dog is fed on flesh from which the juice has been extracted he becomes emaciated after a time, toxic symptoms develop, and death rapidly follows. Skeletal changes characteristic of osteoporosis and osteomalacia are found upon postmortem examination. The extraction of the salts of the flesh causes death. Captive lions were long fed inadequate flesh diets and they failed to breed.

It is well to keep in mind that the different organs of the body differ in their amino acid content. Not merely every species of animal, but also within each animal, every organ has its own peculiar kind of protein. For this reason, the different organs of the animal body are not equally complete or "valuable" as sources of amino acids. I would especially call attention to the low value of muscle meat, the kind of flesh food most commonly eaten.

One advocate of flesh eating deplores the fact that "some patients are unfortunately averse to eating entrails. Entrails, like liver, kidneys, heart, spleen, etc.," he says, "are extremely rich in certain vitamins and other valuable constituents and their regular use in the diet is to be greatly encouraged." To receive all the value of the flesh it is necessary to eat the whole animal and those who are going to consume flesh should not balk at eating the guts. Squeamish flesh-eaters who will eat a cow, but refuse to eat a cockroach are a joke. If the cockroach were as big as the cow, they would cut off, a sizable chunk of its flesh and eat it with gusto. These fastidious carnivores who make grave yards of their stomachs and bury the carcasses of dead animals in them (the corpse eaters) should keep ever in mind that others of their kind in other parts of the world, eat grasshoppers, snails, bees, snakes, ripened (rotten) poultry, rats, mice, cats, dogs, skunks, etc. Poor, degraded scavengers that you are, why be so squeamish? It is not necessary, however, in eating your animals, that you eat the unvoided feces in the colon, as you do in eating oysters whole.

Let me again emphasize that in practical dietetics, we are not concerned with the relative value of specific proteins, nor with the relative value of particular protein foods, but with the total value of the protein contained in our customary diet. And, not with proteins, alone, but with the total diet. We cannot live on proteins alone. We need, besides proteins, carbohydrates, fats, minerals, vitamins. We need, not merely amino acids, but amino acids in ideal combinations with other indispensable substances—minerals, vitamins, carbohydrates—such as only plants can supply. These other substances are essential to the full utilization of protein. Animal proteins are not ideally combined with these other substances. The most ideal substances for both animal and human nutrition (this is true even for the carnivores) and the most ideal blends of these substances are to be found in the spare-products of plants.

There are no amino acids in the proteins of flesh that the animal did not derive from the plant; there is no amino acid in the protein of flesh that the human animal cannot also derive from the plant. The whole question involved in our proposition for consideration is best stated thus: *Is meat, as a whole, superior to vegetables as food?* In answering this question, more factors must be taken into consideration than proteins. In addition to the other food essentials, it is also necessary to take into account the time element. No short time experiment will suffice. The effects of a total flesh diet for a period of generations must be considered.

It may be objected that an exclusive flesh diet is not advocated. I am aware that there are few advocates of such a diet for man. But it is still true that the alleged superiority of a flesh diet can be tested only by employing a flesh diet.

As the final fact for our consideration, let us note that, the animal organism is *incapable of synthesizing amino acids out of raw materials*. This is to say that the animal cannot take the elements of soil, air and water and synthesize amino acids from these. The plant alone possesses the synthesizing power to take the raw materials of earth and make amino acids of them. The animal, then, is either directly or indirectly dependent upon the plant for its amino acids. All amino acids contained in animal proteins, whether those of flesh, eggs or milk, are of plant origin. The cow derives the amino acids contained in milk largely from the weeds, grasses and seeds that she eats; the steer derives the amino acids contained in its flesh from the same sources and from the grains fed "him" while fattening "him." The hen eats grasses, grains, insects and worms from which she derives the amino acids contained in her eggs. The worms and insects which she eats derived their amino acids from vegetable sources. If you eat steak, veal, mutton, lamb, venison, poultry, fish or any other type of flesh food, you do not derive any amino acids from these sources that were not derived by the animals eaten from the plant kingdom. If you drink milk or eat cheese or eggs or any other type of animal food, the amino acids in these foods were derived by the hen, cow or goat from the plant foods she ate. Man is equally capable of securing amino acids from plant foods. Bull-beef and boar-steak are not the only sources of amino acids. Indeed, as we shall see, they are not the best sources of these indispensable food factors.

Plant Proteins

CHAPTER VI

In *Science From an Easy Chair*, second series, p. 173, Sir E. Ray Lancaster, F.R.S., says: "Many vigorous and muscularly well-developed populations in other lands thrive on exclusively vegetable food." This is a statement of fact; not theory. It is not only a fact today, but it has been a fact as far back as recorded history extends and there is archeological and anthropological evidence that it was a fact for long periods of time before written memorials were made.

These peoples are not ethical vegetarians; they are not scientific vegetarians; they have not become vegetarians for the sake of their health; they are not religious vegetarians; they have simply been vegetarians for ages and vegetarianism seems to them the normal and natural order of eating. To such peoples, the theory that vegetable proteins are inadequate, that they are not capable of sustaining growth and development in man, would seem to be as ridiculous as in fact it is. Many centuries of practical experiences by such peoples living on diets containing no animal foods, or of peoples living on diets containing but little animal foods, have certainly demonstrated that satisfactory body-building and maintenance are fully possible without the use of flesh or other sources of animal foods. It should be observed that many of these peoples do not have milk animals and they do not keep poultry for egg production.

The biological value of proteins depends upon their possession of sufficient quantities of the *essential amino-acids,* which cannot be synthesized by animals. The method of determining their value is by feeding experiments upon rats. As the amino-acid requirements of man and rats are different, these experiments do not give dependable results when applied to man. As Prof. Hindhede says: "If one wants to discover the best food for rats, experiments with these animals are the proper ones. But if one wishes to find the best diet for man, one can hardly escape using men for the experiment. Rat experiments may give some hints, but one cannot draw correct conclusions from them."

Rats are of much more rapid growth than man and their amino-acid requirements are correspondingly different. A protein that is adequate for an animal of slow growth may easily prove to be inadequate for one of rapid growth. The more enlightened writers on diet realize that dogmatism based on conclusions arrived at through experiments on rats is very unwise.

It must not be overlooked, also, that the biological value of proteins is usually determined by feeding purified proteins to rats that are being fed a diet that is otherwise free of proteins. It should be kept in mind that the value of proteins is not determined solely by their content of the essential amino acids, but, also, partly by their association with vitamins and minerals. For even a high grade protein cannot sustain life and growth in the absence of a sufficient supply of vitamins and minerals. It is true, on the other hand, that nature never provided isolated proteins. The natural foods eaten by man all possess more or less complex mixtures of proteins. There are numbers of proteins that, when isolated and fed in *pure* form, are incapable of sustaining life and growth, some of them do not even provide for body maintenance. But this is rarely true of the protein mixtures contained in natural foodstuffs. For example, milk contains two proteins, the soya bean contains two proteins, maize contains two proteins; wheat contains two proteins, etc., etc. Now it so happens that, one protein in a food, when isolated and fed in *pure* form to an animal, may prove to be inadequate, whereas, the two proteins in the food, when fed together, prove fully adequate. It is also true that man lives upon a wide variety of protein-containing foods and a deficiency in the protein of one food is compensated by an adequate supply of the lacking amino-acid in one of his other foods.

Prof. Thomas B. Osborne, Ph.D., Sc.D., Research Chemist in the Connecticut Agricultural Experiment Station and Research Associate of the Carnegie Institute, Washington, D. C., spent years and carried out innumerable experiments to determine the precise nature and value of the different proteins. In *The Vegetable Proteins,* he says: "No seed is known which does not contain several different proteins, and in every case examined it has been found that seeds containing a protein deficient in one or more amino-acids also contain another protein in which these amino-acids are present. It is therefore obvious that we cannot conclude that because a considerable part of the protein isolated from a given seed fails to meet the nutritional requirements of a growing animal that the mixture of protein in the entire seed is inferior." Thus, he concludes, after experimenting with barley, oats, rye and wheat, using the whole grain, "that the total protein of each of these seeds is more efficient than has generally been supposed."

Discussing this very point, Prof. E. V. McCollum says: "In practical dietetics neither animals nor man are restricted to a single protein as a source of their necessary amino-acids. Hence, data upon the nutritive value of individual proteins are actually of less utilitarian value than those of the supplementary relationships between such dietary essentials."

There is no single article of food found in all nature that is adequate in every essential nutrient factor, at least not for man, so that most of the experimenting with individual articles of food, instead of determining the adequacy of a given diet, is more or less wasted effort. Most fruits are deficient in calcium, most green leaves contain an abundance of calcium. Nobody lives on fruit alone, so the calcium deficiency of fruits is supplemented by the calcium richness of green leaves.

Regarding the supplementing of each other that occurs when proteins from different sources are eaten, and this is the general rule throughout the animal and human worlds, Dr. J. C. Drummond, Professor of Biochemistry, London University, said in his Harben Lectures, 1942: "It seems clear from the work of the past ten or fifteen years that the mutually supplementary effect of the proteins from cereals, roots and leafy vegetables is such as to provide an excellent amino-acid blend for tissue construction and maintenance. Of course we should have realized this quite clearly from the records of vegetarian peoples, which are quite convincing in this respect."

In this connection Prof. Sherman says that certain experiments "indicate that the nutritive values of legume proteins may in some cases be restricted by their low cystine content, but that this may be readily supplied from other sources." This simply means that the eating of some other food which contains ample cystine renders the total protein intake fully adequate. If we were confined to legumes (excepting peanuts and soya beans) as a source of proteins, we would receive inadequate proteins; but, inasmuch as we are never so restricted, the dangers of protein inadequacy are more imaginary than real. The vociferous advocates of carnivorism have created this bogey out of whole cloth.

It should also be noted that the biological value of a protein is partially determined by other food factors that are present, or absent from the food eaten. For example, it is well known that the utilization of proteins depends upon the presence in the diet of adequate vitamins. Protein assimilation is also increased by an abundance of bases in the diet and it is reduced by their absence or by the presence of too much acid-forming materials. For full utilization of the proteins in any food, the total diet must be adequate in all essentials. This requirement is often lacking in experimental diets, in which many of the food substances used are purified. They must, at least, be deprived of their proteins when the adequacy of a particular isolated protein is being tested, and the very process of extracting their proteins from them also extracts other essentials therefrom.

No one doubts that animal foods can provide adequate amino-acids. This is especially true of eggs, which, as Prof. McCollum says "have a higher nutritive value than any other source of protein known," but it is also true of the flesh of animals, providing one eats the whole animal and does not confine oneself to the muscle meat only. As we do not live upon amino-acids alone, the amino-acid adequacy of a food is not enough to recommend it to us as a superior food. Flesh is deficient in certain vitamins and minerals for which the vegetable kingdom constitutes the best source. Few carnivorous animals, and these consume the whole body of their prey, drinking the blood also, live upon an exclusive flesh-food diet.

As regards purity, stability and reliability plant substances offer the animal proteins and carbohydrates that are superior to those derived from flesh foods. Dr. S. Henning Balfrage says in *The ABC of Food* that flesh foods "contain substances which the body cannot use and which have to be got rid of as waste materials by the liver and kidneys." The fact that flesh foods contain waste products (end-products of animal metabolism which are held up in the tissues at the time of death, plus the products of undetected putrefaction) puts an unnecessary strain upon the human excretory system. It should be noted, in this connection, that in middle aged adults perfectly normal kidneys are the exception rather than the rule.

Among fruits known in this country, the avocado is richest in protein. Good California varieties contain 3.39% protein which is equal to milk in the amino acids essential to the promotion of growth and repair of tissue. Its carbohydrate content being only 2.97% is very low and is made up of sugar and cellulose. One percent of its carbohydrate is in the form of invert sugar. The avocado is rich in a very tasty, emulsified oil which is 93.8% percent digestible. The mineral content of its edible portion runs about 1.18 percent, including ample proportions of the bases calcium, potassium, magnesium and sodium. Copper and manganese are present in smaller quantities. Of vitamins the avocado contains liberal supplies of several of these. It is a good source of *Thiamin* (B_1) and *Riboflavin* (B_2, or G) and is a fair source of A and C (ascorbic acid.)

It will be noted that the protein content of the avocado is a little higher than that of cow's milk, the food supplied by nature for calves during their period of most rapid growth. This protein is ideally combined with vitamins and minerals which enable us to utilize the protein.

Nuts are of such great importance as sources of high grade proteins that I shall devote a separate chapter to them. At this point it need only be said that many of them are richer in protein than flesh foods and that the proteins of practically all nuts (the hickory nut being an exception) are fully equal in amino acid content to flesh. They are certainly a part of the normal diet of man, whereas, flesh is certainly not.

The proteins of legumes and cereals are, in general inadequate, but consumed with an abundance of green vegetables, containing small amounts of high grade proteins, their inadequacies are compensated for. Pigs, rats and other animals fed on grains are able to rear their young, provided the grains are supplemented with an abundance of green fodder. Under natural conditions, grain eating animals, including birds, do not live exclusively on grains, but manifest a peculiar fondness for tender, young greenstuff, which they eat in abundance. On the whole, cereals and legumes are not among the best foods for man, but their relative cheapness and their year around abundance make them useful for the low income groups, providing, of course, they are eaten dry, in proper combinations and with an abundance of raw green vegetables.

The soya bean, which is a rich source of protein of high biological value, is best eaten in the young or green state or as soy sprouts. Young soy sprouts are very tasty and make a fine dish of themselves or an excellent addition to a vegetable salad.

Among the legumes, the peanut is possessed of a rich store of protein of high biological value—this is to say, of an adequate protein. Known also as the ground pea, ground nut and goober, it grows under ground. Its mineral content is made up to a large extent of phosphoric acid and the combination of starch, protein and phosphoric acid makes it a highly acid-forming food. Nonetheless, if eaten with an abundance of green vegetables and not combined with other proteins or carbohydrates, it forms an excellent food. It should, of course, be eaten raw and unsalted and should be well chewed. Roasted and salted peanuts and peanut butters are very poor foods.

Depending upon soil, climate, location, variety and other factors, perhaps not clearly known, the composition of the peanut varies greatly. The proportion of protein runs 25 to 35 percent; fat 50 to 55 percent. The average of over two thousand analyses shows the following composition: water 7.9; protein, 30.0; fat, 50.0, starch and cellulose taken together, about 12.0, minerals, 2.9. Taking into account the fact that the protein of edible flesh averages only about twenty percent, it is easy to see that it would be easy to over eat on peanuts.

If roasted, swallowed half chewed, or combined with starches and other protein foods, the peanut will be digested with difficulty. Like all such foods, it is packed with minerals and vitamins and contains a very tasty oil that is superior to animal fat for human use.

Sunflower seed have long been used as a staple article of diet in Russia and the Balkans and by other peoples. The American Indians had used them for a long period of time before Columbus discovered these Western continents. The Russian soldier is reported to eat them in great quantities. They are a rich source of protein of high biological value, being richer in protein than most meats, eggs and cheese, as well as rich sources of other valuable food properties. Their rich, nut-like flavor is very palatable, while they are easily digested. The yellow, sweet sunflower oil, when expressed from the seed, is considered the equal of olive oil and almond oil for table use.

These seed contain more oil than the soy bean. Varying with the different varieties, sunflower seed contain 27 to 32 percent oil, based on total weight, as compared to 19 percent for soy beans. Sunflower meal tops the list of vegetable concentrates with 52.7 percent protein. The percentage of protein is lower in the whole seed.

As a source of vitamin D, sunflower seed are superior to cod-liver oil, which has many objectionable features and effects. In addition to vitamin D, these seed are richer in the B complex than an equivalent amount of wheat germ and also contain vitamins E and K. They contain liberal amounts of calcium, phosphorus, silicon, magnesium and flourine as well as "trace minerals" and lecithen.

All of this is by way of saying that sunflower seed not only contain liberal amounts of high grade protein, but that they contain them in ideal association with other food factors essential to the utilization of the proteins. As we have previously learned, proteins are useable only in association with other food factors.

It is now proposed to use the oil of the sunflower in the production of oleomargarine, salad dressings, cooking oils and soaps. The meal, we read, can be used as live stock food. Thus again, we have an example of the way in which foolish man, under carnivorism and capitalism, perverts every good thing to a wrong use. Unfortunately for the general public, this excellent food with a very delightful flavor is so high in price that few can afford it as a regular article of diet. Two dollars a pound is too much for anybody to pay for any food. Certainly if they can be produced in Russia and the Balkans so cheaply that the peasants can afford to use them as a staple article of diet, they can be produced in this country much cheaper than they now are. They can be made available for everyone.

Nuts

CHAPTER VII

A source of high grade proteins that is commonly overlooked by experimenters and by the foes of the vegetarian diet, is nuts. Prof. Sherman says: "The nut proteins, in so far as they have been investigated, have shown an amino-acid make-up rather similar to that of the proteins of meat and fish." Dr. Kellogg says: "It is interesting to note that of the several classes of plant foods nuts contain the best protein . . . a study of the relative protein content of nuts, milk and meat shows that, pound for pound, the almond, beech-nuts, and walnut contain on an average as much protein as does meat, and five times as much as is found in milk . . . The chestnut, the filbert, the hickory, pecan and pine nut contain on an average as much protein as is found in fish; while the butternut, the peanut and pignolia contain twice as much and 50% more than is found in the best cuts of meat."

In nature there are many animals of much more rapid growth than man that depend upon nuts as their chief source of protein supply. The amazing strength and soundness of the teeth of these animals that gnaw through the hardest and thickest of nut shells, should make clear, also, that such foods are excellent with which to build and maintain good teeth. The shell of the hickory nut, for example, is very thick and of almost flint-like hardness, yet the squirrel has no difficulty in getting the nut-meat from within.

Rich in protein of high biological value, packed with minerals and vitamins and savored by nature so that they appeal to the gusttory sense of man, such nuts as the pecan, walnut, almond, Brazil nut, pignolia, etc., are not only valuable additions to our diet, but they form a part of the normal diet of the *cheirotheria*. They are not substitutes for flesh food—flesh food is the substitute.

The value of protein food is not to be determined solely by the percentage of protein which it contains, nor yet by the richness of its proteins in the essential amino acids, but by the value of its total food content. Nuts are fairly rich in starches and sugars, are three to four times as rich in mineral salts as flesh and even milk, contain far more vitamins than flesh, while nut albumen is easily assimilated and does not form uric acid. Nuts are rich in fat, which, like that of milk, is in a state of emulsion—that is, ready-made, prepared, or pre-digested, as it were, for circulation through the lymphatic system. If eaten in compatible combinations they are easily digested.

The nut is hermetically sealed within its protecting shell until we are ready to use it, so that it is not subject to contamination. It is doubly protected by the skin over the kernel. Indeed, in some nuts, this inner casing is charged and doubly charged with substances that are so deadly to all forms of bacterial and microscopic life that nothing can touch it or even come within range of its influence without instant destruction. The skin covering the kernels of some of our best nuts is poisonous to man, and must be removed before the nut is eaten. So far as is known, these nut skins are not fatal to man, but they are best removed.

In the green or unripe state of nuts, their flavor is such as to prevent us from eating them. Indeed, the outer shells which encase the nuts also protect against depradation by squirrels or other animals. Tannic acid is common to these outer shells and, indeed, is present in many of the unripe nuts. The acorn, for example, is loaded with raw tannic acid.

Thus nuts supply everything that we can get from flesh foods, in better form, better condition, cleaner, more easily used, and without the risk of eating diseased flesh. Our food animals are fed and cared for in such a manner that they are frequently diseased at the time the butcher batters in their skulls with his pole axe and cuts their throats, to provide the carnivore with "delectible" roasts, steaks and chops. Nuts are not only our very best sources of proteins and fats, but they supply these in ideal combinations with other food factors that are essential to their utilization.

It is not my intention, in this chapter to attempt to discuss all nuts. Instead, I intend briefly to notice only those nuts with which we in America are most familiar. There are nuts in other parts of the world that we know little or nothing of. The immense tropical forests of the Amazon and South American rivers, a region as large as the entire Mississippi Valley, is thickly wooded with many varieties of nut trees. Future generations will doubtless find an inexhaustible supply of the finest and most concentrated foods in these forests, which are far superior to flesh and other animal foods in nutritive and hygienic value. Present generations tend to neglect nuts and our orthodox authorities on nutrition behave often as though nuts do not exist. Let us look at our most common nuts in alphabetical order.

Almond:—Here let me correct a serious error in our common acid-alkaline food tables, and in the writings on diet. It has been said that the almond is an alkalinizing nut. Later research has proved this to be an error. While it does carry an unusually high percentage of alkaline minerals, it is low in potassium, one of the most important of these, and is high in phosphorus, highest of any product of the vegetable kingdom, which would carry it over to the acid side of the scale. This by no means indicates that this fine nut should be avoided; but it does mean that it should be eaten with green things with which it agrees, in order to make it available as food and counteract its acidity.

The skin of the almond should always be removed. It is one of those nuts referred to previously as being self-protecting; and the chemical elements that protect it are of such strongly *astringent* qualities as to be unfit for our use. Blanching, or removing the skins, is very easily done by merely throwing the shelled nuts into hot water. After a minute or two, remove the nuts and wipe off the skins.

An average analysis of almonds shows: Water, 6.00; protein, 24.00; fats, 54.33; carbohydrates (no starch), 10.00; cellulose, 3.00; mineral salts, 3.00.

Many almonds bought in open market have been sulphur-treated. These should be avoided. While the sulphuring is intended to blanch the shells and make them of uniform color, the sulphur frequently penetrates to the kernel, rendering it unfit for food. Buy your almonds and other nuts from sources which you know are proof against the temptations of commercial fraud.

The Brazil-nut or "Nigger-toe" of our childhood, stands high in nutritional value. It is high in fats, and rich in calcium and magnesia. In spite of this latter fact, it is among the acid nuts, due to its high protein content. The Brazil-nut should be blanched, and simply must be thoroughly chewed.

Here is a good average analysis: Water, 4.8; protein, 17.2; fat, 66.00; carbohydrates (mostly sugar), 5.7; cellulose or fibre, 3.0; mineral salts, 3.3.

The Cashew:—This nut is rapidly growing in popularity because of its very attractive flavor and low acidity. Technically it is not a nut, but the seed of a fruit known as the Cashew Apple, which, unlike the seed of any other fruit, grows outside and at the lower end of the "apple."

Because of two little-known acids, cardol and anacardic, which "burn" the mouth and throat, and are quite toxic, the cashew cannot be eaten in its natural raw state. These acids are readily dissipated by low heat. The cashew must be toasted, and the skin removed.

This nut has a flavor peculiar to itself, and should be eaten with green vegetables to be fully appreciated. Never under any circumstances should it be eaten with bread, nor at the same meal with any kind of starch. It is a delightful food, and supplies plenty of first-class protein, although lower in quantity than most nuts. Thus far no satisfactory analysis of the cashew has been made.

The Chestnut:—Although called a nut, looks like a nut, feels like a nut, has a shell like a nut but much thinner than most, the chestnut is shown by analysis to be much more nearly related to the starchy grains than to any of the nuts. Almost as many people, the world over, live principally upon bread and other foods made from chestnut-flour as upon that made from any kind of grain. This is particularly true in the south of France, in the island of Corsica, Asia Minor, the Caucasus, and Northern Africa, while it is an important part of the diet in Italy and Spain. While chestnut trees grow wild in many of the more mountainous parts of the United States, the native production is small, and most of the nuts used here are imported. In Italy it affords one of the principal foods of the workers or peasants. In Switzerland and Germany it also is very widely used. In the countries mentioned the chestnut largely takes the place of *cereal grains* and this is believed by many to be greatly to the advantage of the people since, while the carbohydrate content is much higher than in grains, a greater part of that element is in the form of sugar.

Analysis of the chestnut shows it to contain: Water, 6.0; fats, 8.0; protein, 10.0; carbohydrates (mostly starch), 70.0 (more than double the starch-content of flour made from winter wheat); cellulose, 3.0; minerals, 2.4. Chestnut starch is much more nearly soluble than that of grains. Naturally, the reaction in the body is to decrease the alkaline reserve. We must think that the good health of people who subsist to so great an extent upon chestnuts depends upon an active outdoor life and the consumption of large quantities of uncooked vegetables and fruits.

Cocoanut:—This nut ranks high as a food for man. One of our best known and most freely-used nuts, the cocoanut, like the melon, is much better eaten alone than in the terribly incompatible mixtures in which it is usually eaten. Taken with vegetable salads and cooked green vegetables it digests best; but with starches or sugar, this includes honey, it digests with difficulty. Correctly eaten, alone or with vegetables as mentioned, both the meat and the milk are fine foods for children as well as adults. In countries of which it is a native, the cocoanut makes up just about the complete bill-of-fare of millions of people living in a state of nature.

An average analysis of the cocoanut reveals the following: Water, 3.5; protein, 6.3; fat, 57.4; carbohydrate, sugar and fibre, 31.5; organic salts, 1.3. The minerals are chiefly phosphorus and potassium, with small amounts of sodium, calcium, manganese, and iron. So far as known, it is much the safest course to class the cocoanut with the acid-formers, and balance it with green vegetables. Note that it is not a high protein food, but is abundant in carbohydrates. Its protein is fully adequate.

The Hickory-nut:—The hickory is strictly an American nut. It was used by North American Indians as a principal article of diet. The forests were full of seventeen varieties of hickory trees, until the early settlers, then as now completely ignorant of foods and their value, chopped them down by thousands for fuel, to build rail fences and to form the wooden parts of many implement and machines.

One impediment in the restoration of the Hickory-nut to popularity is its thick, hard shell, quite hard to crack, but that same shell protects the contents perfectly against any sort of contamination.

One of the best of hickories is known as "Hale's Paper Shell." The tree reaches large size, about two feet in diameter and up to seventy-five feet high. The nuts are very large, the shell thinner than that of many pecans, the kernels full, plump and most tasty, having the very rare quality among nuts of keeping several years without becoming rancid.

An average analysis of the seventeen varieties shows the following: Water, 3.7; protein, 15.15; fat, 68.00; carbohydrates (almost all sugar), 12.00; and mineral matter, 2.0. The protein, as is usual with nuts, is of a very high order and, also as usual, this nut requires to be completely masticated and should be eaten with greens only.

The Pecan:—In this country the pecan is one of the most popular of the better nuts. Harter says: "One can live a full life, amply nourished, upon an exclusive diet of pecans and fruits. This is not theory, but an actual fact, demonstrated by members of the League, including the writer. The fatty elements of this nut are more easily assimilated by the human body than any other obtainable."

Once the chief article of food eaten by the Indians, who stored enormous quantities for winter the protein-content of the pecan, while ample for body-needs, is lower than that of most nuts, but it yields the highest percentage of readily usable fat of any of them. Here is an average analysis: Water, 3.5; protein, 13.0; fat, 70.8; carbohydrates (mostly sugar), 8.5; cellulose (fibre), 3.7—just enough "roughage" to favorably influence bowel movement; organic mineral salts, 1.5.

Splendidly protected by its shell from all sorts of contamination, the pecan is ideal. One precaution is necessary; buy your pecans in their shells; and by all means avoid the brightly red-dyed and glossy kernels frequently offered for sale.

The Pignolia or Pine Nut:—There are many varieties of this so-called nut, which is not really a member of the true nut family, although so highly esteemed as such. It actually is the seed of a tree, the stone pine; but has been used as a nut-food from earliest recorded time. It probably was taken up as food by primitive man. This nut comes to us in America from Italy and Southern France, and was popularized through the enterprise of the Morrow nut specialists. It is of a very soft texture; the toothless grandsire can manage it very well; its slightly turpentine flavor may be removed by heating slightly without roasting.

This nut has the highest percentage of protein of any natural food; takes the place of the finest of meats, and a very small portion of it supplies all that the body needs of protein and fats. Chewed to cream, as all nuts should be, the pignolia is very easily digested.

The average of a number of analyses shows the following contents: Water, 6.4; protein, 33.9; fat, 49.4; carbohydrates (simple sugar), 6.0; organic salts, 3.4. The mineral salts are made up largely of calcium, magnesium and iron; and yet, because of its high protein content, the pignolia still ranks as an acid-former.

The Pistachio:—This is one of the very finest nuts, excelling all others in some particulars, most of which are far too little known outside their country of origin. The pistachio comes from Syria.

The kernel of the pistachio is shaped somewhat like a small almond, is greenish in color (the more pronounced the color the better the nut) and has a mild but distinct flavor. This nut, although high in protein, has been found to be *non-acid*, inclined to be alkaline-forming when digested, and its fat-content is very easily digested and assimilated. One peculiarity of this nut is that it contains no indigestible cellulose or fibre; it is all food. Broadly the pistachio contains: Water, 4.2; protein, 22.5; fat, 54.5; carbohydrates (largely, simple sugar), 16.0; organic mineral salts, 3.0.

The Walnut:—Included under this species we have our own native Black Walnut and Butternut, and the imported nut commonly called the English Walnut, although it is not native to the British Isles, but to France and Italy.

The meat of the Black Walnut is far superior to that of either the butternut or the so-called English nut, having a peculiarly full, rich "nutty" flavor. Compared with it, the English nut is "flat, stale and unprofitable," yet to most people the word "walnut" means the English variety only.

A comparative analysis of these three varieties shows:

	Black	*English*	*Butternut*
Water	2.5	2.5	4.5
Proteins	27.5	18.5	27.9
Fats	56.3	64.5	61.2
Carbohydrates	11.7	12.5	3.4
Cellulose	1.7	1.4	None
Minerals	1.9	1.7	3.0

Other Nuts:—A few nuts that exist in other parts of the world and which are not very well known to Americans are the *Castanopis,* or California chestnut, often thought of as a cross between the oak and the chestnut, and eaten by birds and squirrels; the *Chura,* known as the earth-almond, or earth-chestnut, which grows under ground as does the peanut, and which is a vegetable rather than a nut; the *Queensland nut,* which is indigenous to Australia and resembles the Brazil nut, but much superior in flavor; the *Pilinut* or *Javanese Almond,* which grows in the Philippines, Asia and the East Indies; the *Sapucaia* or *Paradise Nut,* little known in America outside New York and the seaboard cities of the East; the *Sauri,* or tropical butternut, a native of British Guiana and seldom seen in this country. This last named nut is pure white, rich and oily and has a pleasing flavor. This is but a partial list of nuts that it is well that we know exist, even though we do not get to eat them.

All nuts, and especially the almond, must be chewed to a creamy consistency if they are to be well digested. The all too common failure to thoroughly chew nuts is partly responsible for their reputation of being "difficult to digest." Except in the case of those individuals who have no teeth with which to chew their foods, nut butters, nut meats and other such nut preparations, which have lost much of their value through oxidation, should not be eaten. Eat the whole nut, fresh from the shell. It will always be best to buy your nuts in the shell.

While nuts cause far less trouble when eaten with bread or other starches than do flesh foods, it is necessary to emphasize that the protein nuts should never be eaten with starches. Pecans, walnuts, almonds, the Brazil nut, the cashew, etc., should be eaten, not with starches and sugars, nor with other proteins, but with green vegetables for ideal results in digestion. Due to their fat content, their combination with tart fruits will not interfere with protein digestion, but the acids of these fruits will definitely interfere with the digestion of the starch. Eating nuts in incompatible combinations is another reason that they are commonly thought of as difficult to digest.

How Much Protein?

CHAPTER VIII

Ever since it was decided that protein is the most important and most essential part of our food, there has raged a controversy over how much protein a day is required to meet the needs of man. At first, the efforts to determine the amount of protein needed were made by merely striking an average of the amount of protein actually eaten by certain groups of men, who are now known to have been gluttonous eaters. Next, an effort was made to determine the amount of protein needed by experiments on dogs. Imagine, trying to discover the protein needs of man by making tests on dogs!

Without going into the matter of these experiments and measurements, suffice it to say that both of them helped to establish a high protein standard, which, although since repeatedly shown to be much too high, is far from dead, both in lay and in professional thought and practice. Indeed, within the last few years, there is apparent a growing tendency to re-affirm the old high-protein standards established by the earlier investigators.

More than seventy years ago Liebig conceived the idea that albumens and proteins are needed in direct proportion to a man's or woman's activity. He thought that the human body is run on the substances of which its muscles and viscera are composed. Of this notion, Drinkwater says: "If muscles are worn away by exercise of their normal function, according to the old view, it would be like a locomotive having to have its wheels and machinery renewed at the end of each journey, instead of needing simply water and fuel." (*Food in Health and Disease,* London, 1906.)

Following Liebig, Voight declared in 1881 that man requires twenty percent of his daily diet to be protein. A little later Atwater made it twenty-five percent, and Moleschott and Veirordt made it twenty percent. Voight experimented upon dogs in his effort to determine the protein requirements of man.

These standards demanded for the adult, who has ceased growing, 7% to 12% more protein (more tissue building material) than nature herself provides for an infant which doubles its weight in six months and trebles its weight in a year. Not until Lahmann in 1892 appreciated this discrepancy and set about to determine the proportions of protein, carbohydrate, fat and salts in mother's milk, and used this information as a basis for calculation for adult diets, was a really decisive blow struck at the old school of dietetics. Lahmann was an old school physician who had associated himself with Louis Kuhne. He noticed that Kuhne's patients, fed as they were on fruits and vegetables, were not receiving the "required" amounts of protein, but fared well on their low protein diet.

Analyzing the ingredients of dried milk, that is water free milk, he found that the fat, sugar and minerals amounted to 85.5 percent of the whole; the protein present amounted to only 13.5 percent. Thus for a growing baby, producing more tissue daily than does the adult, nature provides a diet, which, apart from water, contains only 13.5 percent of the tissue building material called protein. But relative to the total bulk of breast milk taken by an infant, the protein is really only 1.6 percent, because it is 88 percent water. Only in relation to the ingredients other than water is the amount 13.5 percent. This is said, however, not to be wholly a reliable basis of calculation, because unless we know the adult's activity as compared with that of the baby, we cannot accurately assess the adult's need.

Drinkwater says that "the most strenuous muscular labour does not increase in the smallest degree the metabolism of albuminates (proteins) in the body; it is the non-nitrogeneous alimentary principles, the fats and carbohydrates, whose consumption is increased by muscular activity." It would seem, therefore, that our need in accurately assessing the protein needs of the adult as compared to that of the infant, would be a knowledge of the relative differences in tissue building activity that goes on in the two organisms.

In 1887 Hirshfeld made a series of experiments and placed the protein standard at 47 grains, but the "scientists" rejected his standard. A young man of twenty-four years, Hirshfeld performed heavy labor, weight lifting, mountain climbing, etc., on a diet containing less than half the protein thought to be necessary. He lost neither weight nor strength, while the "nitrogen balance" showed that he did not lose body protein. Hindhede says of his work: "It is strange, indeed, that Hirshfeld's investigations have been permitted by science to drift almost into oblivion. He was a young man (twenty-four) who could make little impression upon the weight of Voight's authority." The low protein standard attracted little attention until after Horace Fletcher startled the "scientists" out of their lethargy.

Chittenden in 1904 protested against the over-consumption of protein and established three ounces daily as the average adult requirement. It was not, however, until a little later, when it was shown that the amount of urea excreted is by no means proportionate to the activity indulged in, that Liebig and his school, together with the whole of the dietetic conventions that were supported by his ideas, were ultimately shown to be completely false.

We must cease to think of the adult's activities as involving chiefly the expenditure of his protein elements, his tissues, but as the expenditure of his fuel. Compared, therefore, with the protein needs of the growing infant, who is making more tissue daily, those of the adult are very small indeed. Therefore, to make 13.5 percent of the diet of the adult, protein, would be ridiculous.

Lahmann was in favor of conforming to the proportion of milk. This was too high, particularly as he used cow's milk as his standard. Chittenden maintained that "body-weight, health, strength, mental and physical vigor and endurance can be maintained with at least one-half of the protein food ordinarily consumed." He estimated the proportion of protein for the adult at 3.5 percent lower than for the infant, and thought that health could be maintained much more satisfactorily on about 10 percent of protein in the diet than on 20 percent.

It was later found that the estimates of both Lahmann and of Chittenden are much in excess of actual body needs, for active grown men. Boyd, taking flesh as the source of protein, estimated the minimum daily ration of protein requisite to maintain body-weight at 30 grammes, i.e., only 4.65 percent in a total amount of 650 grammes of food. (Vitamins, London, 1923, P. 61.) Ragnar Berg, after making a more accurate investigation, found it to be only 26 grammes, or 4 percent of the total (Vitamins, London, 1923); while Rose, after providing a better supply of bases, found it to be only 24 grammes, or only 3.7 percent. (Vitamins, London).

After carefully surveying all previous estimates and after conscientious experimentation of his own, Berg came to the conclusion that the adult body's need of protein should be calculated on a basis of .58 grammes per killogramme of body weight (Vitamins). Berg concluded that "a supply equivalent to 1 gramme of protein per kil-logramme of body-weight, when a mixed diet is taken . . . provides a margin of safety of from 50 to 100 percent."

Thus a fully grown adult, of say 140 lbs. should consume not more than 2.2 ounces of protein a day—*i.e.*, if he is taking his protein in the form of meat, or cheese, he should not take more than half a pound of beef or curd cheese altogether; or if he is taking it in the form of cod-fish, not more than 7/8 of a pound.

It is obvious that the average full-grown man, even of moderate habits, allows himself a much larger proportion of protein. If he has eggs and bacon for breakfast, these alone, apart from the bread he consumes with them, will provide 3/5 of his daily quota of 2.2 ounces of protein, leaving only 1.6 ounces for his lunch and dinner. Thus, by the time he has his lunch, consisting of a cut from a joint, a chop or a steak, he has consumed more than his quota, and the rest is all excess as far as protein is concerned, quite apart from the bread, potatoes, milk or cereals he may also have had.

Ragnar Berg allows a small increase of protein for reproduction, and in this case proteins of high biological value are essential. But when reproduction is allowed for, it is obvious from the previous figures that the average man who has ceased growing, indulges to excess in those kinds of foods which are body building and which he does not require, and thus, not only deprives his body of other important elements, such as mineral salts and vitamins, but also impedes the combustion of his running fuel. Hindhede reared four athletic and wide-awake children on a diet so low in protein that it has been said "it would frighten a school teacher into blind staggers."

Nixon, who is no vegetarian and has no bias in favor of vege-tarianism, writing in January 1934 said that 100 grams of protein daily (*i.e.*, 3.527 ounces or nearly 1/4 lb.) is "the average require-ment for physical and mental activity and for fertility, 50 grams of which should be "first class protein" by which he means meat, eggs, cheese, including fish. This is the amount of protein he regards as sufficient for a young man in his prime when reproductive powers are at their zenith. This means that one-half the young adult's daily protein consumption should be high grade proteins. Vegetarians would use as proteins of high biologic value nuts, peanuts, avocadoes, soy beans, bananas, and green vegetables.

In my own work, I have watched hundreds of men, women and children make steady (often rapid) gains in weight and strength following lengthy fasts, while consuming less than half the protein daily that is supposed to be required. I have reared children and supervised the rearing of many more on a diet containing far less protein than the prevailing standards call for and the healthiest and finest developed children I have seen have been these very children. My feeding program comforms closely to the standard established by the Swiss experiment, an account of which follows.

Some recent experiments made in Switzerland should go far to settle a long-sought-for solution to the problem of how much protein is required daily for an individual. Unlike most experiments that have been made in an effort to solve this problem, this experiment was made on human beings and on large numbers of them. If its conclusions do not agree with the findings of the rat-pen dietitians, this will merely be hard on the boys in the rat-pens.

The British Association for the Advancement of Science was addressed at its regular meeting about two years ago by a Swiss speaker, Prof. A. Fleisch. He told the assembled scientists that experiments carried out with scientific thoroughness on 4,000,000 people in Switzerland showed that the amounts of calories, proteins and fats formerly considered essential in civilized countries were utterly unnecessary. He asserted, on the basis of these experiments, that the United Nations minimum standard of 2,400 calories a day is too much and that 2,160 is sufficient for all except heavy manual workers. The conclusion reached through their experiments is that one gramme of protein per kilo (0.035 oz. per 2 1/4 lb.) of body weight is correct. Before the war the protein requirements were supposed to be 100 grammes (3 1/2 oz.). This amount he asserted, was not only unnecessary, but was actually harmful. He said that a large part of the meat and eggs eaten before the war and a large part of the refined fats, sugar and white bread and macaroni could have been replaced by vegetables, fruits and darker bread.

Finally, he said that today, when great nations of the world are suffering from hunger, it is absolute waste to convert large quantities of wheat into eggs, thus losing 90 percent of the nutritive value of the wheat, and to convert tremendous amounts of maize (corn) and barley into fodder (food for cows) and thus lose 75˚ percent of the calories and proteins. This is a direct stab at our traditional but nonetheless foolish agriculture which first raises huge quantities of food for animals, feeds it to the animals, and then feeds man a small percentage of the food value thus converted into animal foods.

It will seem amazing to most of my readers that only about one-half the amount of protein considered necessary before the war is really needed daily by the individual for health and strength. The old high protein standards thus go glimmering through the things that were. No doubt the packers and the poultry men will not like this and a great howl will go up from the rat pens. The radio touts who look after the interests of the meat packing industry will shout themselves hoarse denying the validity of these tests made on men and women instead of rats. Nonetheless, there is but one way to determine the nutritive requirements of man. In dealing with the young, the requirements of a rapidly growing animal and those of an animal of slow growth are very different.

While the efforts of most investigators seem to have been directed to ascertaining minimum protein requirements, it may be debatable as to whether or not this can establish a valid standard for protein intake. It is quite clear, however, that greater sobriety in the matter of nitrogen (protein) ingestion is essential not only to achieve a return to health, but also in order to maintain health at its highest peak at all times and for all purposes. Reinheimer truly says that "nitrogen, the chief ingredient of protein, is universally a good servant, but a bad master." It is well known to physiologists that both fat and protein metabolism depend upon carbohydrate metabolism. There is a delicate balance between carbohydrates and proteins, to which we have to conform—disease and degeneration resulting from failure to conform.

It has been shown that excess nitrogen is detrimental to the capacity for work, while very generally, it is the accumulation of a nitrogen product, *kinotoxin*, in the muscles that is the cause of fatigue. Men are poisoned by excessive protein ingestion. More than any other food factor, excesses of protein foods fill the body with toxins. Indeed, the whole system becomes overcharged with poisonous products of protein metabolism, which the eliminative functions eventually fail to cope with. The calamitous moribundity of a body poisoned by unsuitable and excessive protein is similar to the case of *alimentary anaphylaxis*.

In middle aged adults, perfectly normal kidneys are the exception rather than the rule. By a careful selection of a low nitrogen diet, it is possible to reduce the amount of work required of the kidneys to a level at which they are able to keep the waste products in the blood within normal limits.

We can say, without fear of successful contradiction, that a disproportionately increased amount of protein in the diet, due to the arbitrary addition to the diet of foods rich in protein, such as flesh, eggs, cheese, etc., proves harmful, as a continual excess of protein results in severe disturbances of health. Yet these are the very foods that the advocates of much "high-grade" protein place greatest stress upon. An excess of protein thus provided, (this improperly prepared and wrongly combined), is the source of much trouble.

Fruits, Nuts, Vegetables

CHAPTER IX

In my little book, *Food Combining Made Easy*, I emphasize the fact that man, the archtype of the *cheirotheira*, should develop those frugivorous habits which are common to his anatomical structure and from which he has largely departed in the course of time, due, no doubt, in large measure, to his wanderings since he left his edenic home in the warmer regions. Many naturalists and comparative anatomists, not the least of these being Prof. Thomas Henry Huxley, have shown that man, as a primate, definitely belongs in the class of frugivores rather than in the class of gramivores, omnivores, carnivores, and sapraphytes, but it was Sylvester Graham who strongly emphasized the obvious fact that by as much as man differs from the other frugivores, they stand between him and the other classifications. *Man is the archtype of the frugivores.*

The human constitution is the final umpire before which to arbitrate whatever questions may in any way affect man. Man is a biological, not a chemical unit, and the matter of the normal diet of man should be approached from the biological standpoint. The fact that all the indications afforded us by chemistry, in our choice of nutrients, are of a more or less negative character, renders the biological approach all the more important.

Comparison of the structure of man's own organism with that of the lower creatures nearest to him, certainly condemns his carnivorous practices and brands them as one of those perversions into which he has fallen, perhaps, as a matter of necessity, in some remote past. Cuvier, one of the greatest naturalists of the last century, says: "Man appears to be formed to nourish himself chiefly on roots, fruits, and the succulent parts of vegetables. His hands make it easy for him to gather them; the shortness and moderate strength of his jaws, the equal length of his canine teeth with the others, and the tubular character of his molars, permit him neither to graze, nor to devour flesh, unless such food is first prepared by cooking . . ."—*Regne Animal*, Vol. 1, p. 73.

In the animal kingdom we observe the general characteristics of the granivora, carnivora, frugivora, etc., but also family characters, such as those among mammalia, the cheirotheria, including the bimana and quadrumana of Cuvier, to which man belongs by the analogies and correspondences of his anatomical structure. Those creatures, in their natural state, subsist on fruits and on vegetable products, although like man, they are capable, through a perverted education, of carnivorous habits. Man has, behind, the grinding teeth, teeth fitted for the comminution of grains and roots, and not the scissors teeth of the carnivora; before, the cutting teeth of the frugivora, and those called canine are also of this type. He has none fit for tearing raw flesh, and the grinding motion of the jaw results from the development of the pterygoid muscles peculiar to the gramivora, and essentially differing from the vertical motion which corresponds with the scissors teeth of the carnivora. The length of his alimentary canal is again characteristic, and confirms the former analogies.

It is said that Cuvier definitely settled the question of the dietetic nature of man. While I believe that this assertion is true, although I would not exclude others who have duly considered this matter from due share in the credit for having settled the question as to man's normal mode of nutrition, I know that European and American peoples have been unwilling to accept the answer that has been given. M. Bircher-Benner, M.D., of Switzerland, quotes a European scientist, Dr. Richard Lehne, who sums up his conclusions, after a careful and exhaustive comparative anatomical study, in these words: "Quite apart from the physiological findings of nutritional science, which perpetually alter and are always in an unsettled form, comparative anatomy proves—and is supported by the millions-of-years-old documents of palaeozoology—that human teeth in their ideal form have a purely frugivorous character."

Man's sense of taste does not even now, after many thousands of years of eating flesh, demand flesh and will learn a more exquisite appreciation of the savours of the great variety of fruits, vegetables and nuts in their many and varied artistic combinations, which appeal as much to his eye and nose as to his tongue. The beauty of fruits and their delightful aromas are in striking contrast with the ugliness of a roast and the objectionable odor of a fish market or a butcher shop.

The old medical delusion that fruits are practically devoid of food value still lingers in the minds of millions of people. They think of fruit as a "relish," or as an "appetizer," or as a "dessert." Many people are actually afraid of fruits, a survival of the medical teaching of a few decades ago, that fruits cause many diseases. In striking contrast with this teaching of the medical profession was the practice of many *Hygienists* of that very time of eating nothing but fruit for breakfast. At the same time all of them discarded refined flour products, while most of them eschewed butter and all greasy preparations. They also abstained from tea, coffee, etc., and ate no cakes or pies. They took no drugs and gave none to the members of their families.

"Fruits of love," as Lazarus, an early *Hygienist*, called such fruits as peaches, plums, apples, pears, grapes, oranges, etc., are as abundant in food values as they are packed with delicious savoriness. Lazarus thought the designation "fruits of love" was especially appropriate for those fruits that ripen in the Spring, that is, "during the season of love." It is known that in fruit and date eating natives wounds heal much more quickly than they do in flesh eating Europeans. This would seem to indicate a superiority of the fruit diet over the flesh diet. In my observation of the healing of wounds in domestic carnivores as compared with the healing of wounds in domestic vegetarians, I have noted the carnivores heal less readily. The general effect of plant food on the animal is wholesome and restraining, while flesh foods are disintegrating and accelerating.

Our very existence as civilized peoples depends upon vegetarian or fruitarian fare. Whenever, in the life of a people, agriculture supersedes hunting, the nobler forms of existence and of brotherhood and a reduction of all manners of parasitic nurture, with a diminution of disease and greater physiological perfection follow. There follows, also, the possibility of maintaining greater populations on smaller areas. In his *Mutual Aid*, Kropotkin tells us of savages: "It has been remarked that as soon as they succeed in increasing their regular means of subsistence, they at once begin to abandon the practice of infanticide." It has repeatedly been pointed out that all genuine human wealth has been wrought along the lines of work and cultivation in opposition to vagrancy, depradation and parasitic nurture. Only prejudice and false science are opposed to fruitarianism.

Among graminivorous and frugivorous animals social aggregation is the rule and isolation the exception, while, among the carnivora isolation is the rule and social aggregation the exception. A
predatory life not only calls for greater space on which to secure
sustenance, but the very nature of the life itself literally organizes
into the character of the predatory man or beast, the "spirit" of
conflict and incoherence. Of a life sustained by violence and force,
fraud and force are the natural expressions. The carnivorous habit
of man requires large uninhabited tracts of country to support but
few individuals. Hunting and fishing provide but small quantities
of food as compared to agriculture, from the same expanse of ter-
ritory.

There is every reason to think that the social league of human
brotherhood is broken up when man becomes a beast of prey; so
that each, like the wolf or the tiger, makes his lair apart. On the
other hand, as soon as he seeks to regain his lost purity and re-
nounces his habit of preying, he begins to feel the necessity for
higher forms of social life than are consistent with the parcelling and
incoherence of interests and with the superficial and coarse relations in which the greater number of individuals stand to their fellow men in a predatory existence.

There follows also a more refined and exquisite sensibility of
the various organs of the body, when these are developed under a
vegetable and fruit regimen, which not only adds immensely to the
joys of living, but also multiplies and intensifies our relations with
nature. The ancient tradition that God placed the original human
pair in a Garden of Delight and made of them "keepers of the
garden," takes us back to the period when man, in keeping with
his constitutional nature, lived upon the bountiful produce of nature
without resorting to the killing of animals for food. The delights
of the garden are strikingly unlike the miseries of the slaughter house.

Must we go on getting our food at second-hand through other
animals, instead of taking it, as they do, fresh and fine and full of
life, from the bountiful gardens and orchards of nature? Must we
forever violate the plainly obvious constitutional nature of man in
our eating habits and live upon foods that are but poorly fitted to
satisfy our nutritional requirements? I plead not for the animal
only, as is the habit of ethical vegetarians, but for man also, who is

hurt by this divorce from his normal way of life. He inflicts more
suffering and woe upon himself by his departure from the path of
biological rectitude than he measures out to his food animals. Only
by a return to the plant kingdom as the source of his food supply,
can he hope to be superiorily nourished.

Upon examination we find that we have many foes, as well as
many friends, in the world of plants, and that much of the vigor of
life depends upon using plants in obedience to the laws and instincts of organic life, not in obedience to the fictional laws of false
science or *therapeutics*. To the *Hygienist* it is a never ceasing source
of amazement that poisonous plants have always been employed as
medicines (healing agents), while the nutritive plants have rarely
been invested, by the medicine men, ancient and modern, with any
so-called healing virtues. If a plant is sufficiently poisonous to be
deadly, so that arrows dipped in its juices mean sure death to whom-
soever they strike, that plant and that poison is a *medicine*. The
whole of the ancient and modern herbal practice consists in employing as *medicines*, poisonous plants. A non-poisonous plant has no
curative powers. This practice is as absurd as the practice of the
man who abstains from tomatoes, oranges, etc., lest their use give
him rheumatism, but who uses tobacco with the thought that is is
harmless, perhaps, even, beneficial.

Carnivorism

CHAPTER X

There was an Australian *aborigine* who justified his act of killing and roasting his wife by saying: "she tasted good." The cannibal goes out and hunts, pursues and kills another man and proceeds to cook and eat him precisely as he would any other game. There is not a single argument nor a single fact that can be offered in favor of flesh eating that cannot be offered, with equal strength, in favor of cannibalism. Indeed, cannibalism is so rampant among carnivorous animals and men that it would not be difficult to show that flesh eating leads directly to eating one's own kind. Paleontologists tell us that some of the stone age peoples had sunk into cannibalism. Cannibalism has been practiced by highly civilized peoples and is far from unknown among modern civilized peoples.

The carnivora fail to provide a criterion for what constitutes wholesome nutrition. It is certain that they do not obtain from their ill-gotten fare the nutritive "stimulation" requisite for stability. It is well known that a high infant mortality obtains among carnivora. This indicates a serious decline of viability among these animals.

Carnivorous animals are debarred, by their morbid habits, from first-hand supplies of vitamins and from the indispensable juices of fruits and vegetables and their ingredients and, consequently, they develop increasing metabolic abnormalities. In place of the nobler foods, predaceous species are forced to be content with inferior products, and while these are not prejudicial to bulk and numbers, they are prejudicial to integrity, stability and progressive development. Indeed, the predominance of inferior physiological values frequently means additional "stimulation" of a deteriorating nature, producing increasing degeneration. The animals preyed upon very generally represent the offal of life—in wild nature generally, sick animals and weak or dead and decaying ones, and in civilization those rendered morbid by domestication and wrong feeding. Carnivora and saprophytes which batten on the offal of terrestrial life—the domesticated pig eating its own excreta, the domesticated chicken eating human and animal excreta, all of them eating dead and decaying flesh—are content with poor food supplies. The appetites of scavengers grow with what they feed upon, so that they tend to eat more and more filth. For the very reason that meat and fish are poor sources of vitamins, it is often suggested that glandular tissue, such as liver, should be added to the diet. But it is known that liver increases, even more than muscle meat, the amount of creatine in the urine.

No wonder they have a high infant mortality and, despite plural births, are relatively few in number in nature. The predacious life unfits them for living. Darwin hinted that the carnivores may improve their chance of life by becoming less carnivorous and said that liability to extinction may be due to "lack of improvement according to the principle of the all-important relations of organism to organism in the struggle for life." This is a faint recognition of the principle of *symbiosis* so fully developed by Herman Reinheimer of England. Extending the thought presented by Darwin, Reinheimer says that "it is in consequence of a neglect of legitimate alimentation that predacious types, setting themselves against the most fundamental and sacred Cosmic laws of assimilation and of division of labor, suffer an obliteration of all normal ratios of life, drifting deeper and deeper into morbidity and parasitism." He views, and I believe, rightly, the insectivore, carnivore, parasite, cannibal, saprohyte, and all other types of predacious plant and animal as pathological types. They do not represent the norm of nature and are each and all steeped in degeneracy and headed for ultimate extinction.

This view is the direct antithesis of that held by the average zoology professor, who, opportunist by profession, seems to delight in picturing the carnivore as representing the very norm and pink of life, thereby expediently justifying our own carnivorous practices. Why, will someone please explain, has man chosen to follow the least virtuous of the animals, the carnivora? Our carnivorous biologists are forever offering up incense to the god of waste. Dry bones and cutlets are all they impute to any creature and these are all they get out of it. There are too many "scientists" who prefer to range themselves on the side of the majority (or on the side of Big Business interests) and to defend conventional views (or defend special interests), rather than range themselves on the side of truth. This procedure assures them popularity and money.

As most flesh foods are deficient in both minerals and vitamins and practically devoid of carbohydrates, and, as most animal fats are regarded as inferior types of fats, even by the defenders of the carnivorous diet, flesh eating is defended almost wholly upon the ground that it is a ready source of superior proteins. It is asserted that flesh proteins are superior to proteins of plant origin, hence preferable to these. It is even asserted, on the basis of recent animal experiments, that animal proteins are absolutely indispensable. The *Hygienist* takes the opposite view.

We hold that the flesh and juices of other animals are, at best, only second-hand foods. The serum and ready-made protein of other animals constitute a danger. It is one of our biological duties to elaborate our own specific proteins out of simple compounds and not to encumber ourselves with the proteins of other animals. Our protoplasm is likely to be impoverished, rather than enriched by predacious feeding, which is easily shown to be pregnant with patho-logical effects. It has been shown that with certain important protein reactions the carnivora behave differently than the herbivora, the latter showing greater powers of synthesis and defense. It is quite true that flesh foods and other animal substances contain some of the residual energies originally derived from the plant, but these are mixed with certain unreliable and often dangerous substances which disturb and deteriorate the primordial values originally derived from the plant.

The unfitness of certain substances for assimilative purposes is manifest by the *anaphylactic* symptoms which so frequently follow their use. Nature, in vetoing certain proteins, chiefly animal, is endeavoring to promote the stability of the species and protect the health of the individual. *Allergy* and *anaphylaxis,* so far from being mysterious, are in reality, due to long standing poisoning of the body by excess or inappropriate protein foods.

Although the assertion is commonly made that animal proteins are more easily digested and more fully assimilated than plant proteins, the phenomena of *anaphylaxis,* so frequently following the ingestion of many animal proteins, suggests that the human digestive system is not adequately equipped for the digestion of the more complex proteins and that the simpler proteins of the vegetable kingdom are best suited to man's digestive abilities. While it does not support my view that the plant proteins are more easily digested than are the animal proteins, the following statement by Professor E. F. Terroine, of the University of Strassbourg and Director of the Institute of General Pathology of the Faculty of Sciences, fails to uphold the popular view. He says: "There are no grounds based upon digestibility for discriminating between proteins according to origin."

My position is that *anaphylaxis* or protein *allergy* is poisoning due to the absorption of but partially digested proteins. This is to say, they are not reduced to amino acids, but are absorbed in more complex form, hence are poisonous. Amino acids are not poisonous, hence should give rise to no *anaphylactic* phenomena.

It is a curious fact that, while flesh-eaters insist that flesh-food is a source of strength superior to plant-foods, they continue to confine themselves largely to muscle-flesh and this is definitely a deficient food. Not only is it deficient, originally, but by the time the cooks have boiled, broiled, baked, fried and otherwise "prepared" it, it is even more deficient. It is deficient, both from its losses in cooking and from its changes while in storage. It is replete with putrefactive poisons as well as with the normal metabolic waste that was held up in the tissues of the animal at the time of death.

The genuine carnivore not only eats the whole body of his prey and drinks his blood, but takes it raw, else would he die from deficiency. In the blood, bones and bone marrow and in the glands of his prey exist the better nutritive portions of the dead animal. With all of this, the beast of prey is forced to supplement his flesh diet, from time to time, with foods of plant origin. If you must eat flesh, why can you not learn from the carnivores and eat it as they do—uncooked and unmixed. These animals never take bread or baked potatoes with their flesh foods. They thus avoid the indigestion that results from such incompatible combinations.

We know that the flesh of animals is not necessary for anyone; that flesh foods are not our best sources of proteins and fats; that everything we get from flesh, except its content of animal waste, its diseased portions and the putrefactive poisons it contains, may be had in better and more usable condition from many other foods, especially nuts. The splendid fitness of octogenarian and nonagenarian vegetarians is enough to cause us to hurl defiance in the teeth of "science," when it so brazenly proclaims the superiority and indispensability of flesh foods.

A glance about us will quickly reveal that the wisest, strongest and most useful, the most beautiful and longest-lived animals are not flesh eaters—the monkeys and apes, the squirrels, rabbits, elephants, sheep, cows, horses, and many others; while those animals that seem to exist only to bedevil and prey are carnivorous—the cats, from the domestic cat, through the leopard and tiger to the lion, the rats, mice, the hyena, and all the rest of the killers. It is with these latter that our expediency-serving biologists would align us.

The fact is that the more carnivorous man becomes, the lower down in the scale of civilization and culture he slides. In lowly organized tribes and communities of men, who live by hunting and fishing, or by gathering such foods and other supplies as are to be had by gathering and picking up, and who do no productive work, the number of parasitic and predatory individuals is necessarily limited by the number of animals of which it is possible to make a prey. Such tribes may be found eating insects, snakes and various other low forms of animal life, including half rotted carcasses. Organisms may resist dissolution in spite of the presence of morbific influences so that these degraded tribes of men continue to survive, but they remain stationary—they make no advance.

In Aug. 1951 Col. Charles Lawrence, executive secretary of the institute of food technologists, issued a statement that worms, slugs and garden snails are excellent sources of protein. He stated that his own favorite dish is pickled Mexican worms bedded on rice. He and other American soldiers, held in a Japanese prison camp after their capture on Bataan, ate worms, land snails, tree lizards and pythons, and thus kept themselves alive. He tells of the men eating wormy rice, worms and all. In an extremity such as these men were in, men will eat anything rather than starve to death, but this seems hardly to be sufficient reason to introduce such articles of diet into the diet of the people when no such extremity exists. The instinct of expediency and the pressure of necessity will always supersede sentiment in the matter of eating, as elsewhere; but when the necessity no longer exists, there is no reason why the expedient should be perpetuated. On the other hand, there is no reason, save that of squeamishness, why the cow eater should not also be a worm or snail or lizard eater.

Flesh eating is frequently defended on the specious plea that if we do not eat the animals they will soon multiply to so great an extent that they will overrun the earth. Whatever may be the truth about this, and it is questionable that such a thing would ever occur, it is a false issue to suppose that man must eat animals in order to prevent an excess in numbers of them. Certainly there are enough carnivores, without the aid of man, if their services are required, to keep down the number of animals. There is no more need for man continuing his carnivorous practices than there is for him to continue those practices that ally him with the scavengers.

It should be known that much of the present propaganda in favor of eating animal foods is motivated by cash supplied by the dairy, poultry, fish and packing industries. Since the ending of World War II, the meat packing industry has been particularly anxious to build up the myth that man cannot be adequately nourished without animal proteins. Many people learned during the war that they could get along with less flesh foods or with no flesh foods at all. These must be recaptured for the meat business. No business likes to lose its customers. One radio pitch man who is very vigorous in his denunciation of vegetarianism and in his insistence that man must eat animal foods, gives away hams over the radio as a means of inducing people to listen to his meat-selling talks. It is well, always, when one of these men begins his talk for flesh-eating, to stop him long enough to ask what he is selling and who is paying his salary. If you know what he is selling and who pays his salary, you may then know what he "thinks" and why he says what he does. "Money talks." It also writes, as Sinclair has shown.

Much of what is called "research" is also motivated by the cash supplied by the meat-packing industry. Experiments are conducted by men of science, the experiments being financed and the scientists being paid for their work with funds provided by the meat industry. Their experiments are carefully "controlled" so that they reveal what the paymaster wants revealed. It should never be forgotten that these men of science may be purchased at a dime a dozen, even in these days of inflation.

Sulphured Fruits

CHAPTER XI

Commercial syrups and certain dried fruits, such as the peach, apple, pear and apricot, are bleached by being subjected to the fumes of burning sulphur. This is the source of the sulphur dioxide that is in them. There are two primary reasons why fruits are treated with sulphur. These are: 1.—The bleaching of the fruit gives them a much more appealing color and appearance so that people, who buy foods by appearances only, buy such foods in greater quantity. 2.—Sulphuring dried fruits enables the producers to put them on the market with a much higher water content—as high as thirty percent. Unsulphured fruits have a water content of only fifteen to twenty percent. The sulphuring of fruits enables the manufacturers to sell more water at a big price per pound.

It used to be asserted that sulphuring kills insects and prevents insects from getting into the fruit. That no self-respecting weavel or other insect will eat sulphured fruits is true, but this is an excellent reason why you should also abstain from eating such fruits. The sulphur dioxide contained in these fruits is a poison that kills insects and injures you.

At present, it is asserted that the sulphuring process preserves certain of the vitamins of the fruit. This is probably only a commercial claim. It is freely admitted that the process does destroy certain of the vitamins.

The sulphurous acid contained in sulphured fruits results in definite and marked physiological injury to the user. As early as 1907 it was shown to damage the kidneys, with the function of which it interferes. It also destroys both red and white blood cells. It is a poison and no poison can be taken into the body without undesirable consequences.

In circular No. 37 issued November 22, 1907, the Government said: "Sulphurous acid in the food produces serious disturbances of the metabolic functions. It adds an immense burden to the kidneys, which cannot result in anything but injury. It impoverishes the blood in respect to the number of red and white corpuscles. It is in every sense prejudicial to health."

In 1911 the Department of Agriculture had a study made by a Board of Consulting Scientific Experts. This study was far from complete and leaves much to be desired. They found that sulphur dioxide in quantities of three-tenths of a gram daily (this amount may be derived from six or eigtht ounces of dried fruit) gives rise, after a period of some months, to symptoms indicating injury. They noted the following symptoms: "increase in uric acid, destruction of white corpuscles, belching of sulphur dioxide gas, teeth 'on edge,' inflammation of the mucous membrane of mouth, symptoms of malaise, headache, backache, sick appearance, nausea, albumenuria, sensation of cold, white color (anemia), dull eyes, listless manner . . ."

The escape of sulphur dioxide from manufacturing plants using this gas destroys the vegetation in the surrounding country and injures man and beast. This is precisely the reason insects refuse to eat sulphured fruits. The poisonous character of this gas is shown by the commission reporting to the Bureau of Mines on its investigation made between June 1913 and September 1914, which stated that the presence of 35 parts of sulphurous acid in 1,000,000 parts of air is harmful to man and that as little as 2 parts of the poison in 1,000,000 parts of air applied for four hours at a time or for ten minutes a day had injurious effects upon plant life and that it lowered the yield of barley studied during the investigation.

Before sulphurous acid can be eliminated from the body by the kidneys it must first be combined with alkalies. It thus robs the body of bases and helps to lower its alkalinity. This is an important objection to the use of sulphured foods of all kinds.

Concentration of attention upon vitamins has resulted in more fallacies being promulgated about food than did the prior concentration upon calories. But, in line with the present vogue, sulphuring of fruits is defended on the ground that it preserves certain of the vitamins in fruits. In the drying process (any drying process) there is a loss of much of the vitamin content of foods. For example, vitamins A and C are lost in the drying process. Niacin and riboflavin (B_2) are not lost to any great extent in the drying process, nor is B_1, except in sulphured fruits. It is asserted that sulphuring of fruits preserves vitamins A and C. But, it is at the same time, admitted that these vitamins are slowly lost in storage. It is contended that the saving of vitamins A and C by the sulphuring process is more important than the loss of B_1 by the same process. And, thus, the poisoning of our dried fruits is seemingly justified. It is, of course, admitted that the effect of drying processes, including the sulphuring process, is variable.

As no one depends upon dried fruits for one's vitamin supply, as fresh fruits and vegetables are far more abundant sources of these foods, even at their best, and as the eating of sulphured fruits results in marked physiological damage, there is simply no justification for the sulphuring practice, except the commercial one. Our ignorant people prefer to buy the white or golden colored fruits to the unbleached kinds—sulphured fruits sell better besides carrying more water.

For years the Bureau of Chemistry, Department of Agriculture of Washington and the dried fruit industry fought each other at great lengths over this matter, but the government never really acted. The Food and Drug Laboratory of the University of California once openly criticized the government for its failure to act. But the sulphur interests and the fruit industry have been powerful enough to prevent the government from acting in the matter.

Not all governments have been so derelict in their duty in this respect. England, France, Germany, Switzerland and Japan placed embargos on American dried fruit "because of the excessive sulphur content." The Department of Agriculture laments that "American dried fruit is now in very considerable disfavor abroad, because the use of sulphur has gone 'entirely too far.'" It is correct to say that this same dried fruit is in complete disfavor among those Americans who know. Only the uninformed consume sulphured fruits.

Oxidation of Foods

CHAPTER XII

Oxidation is the union of oxygen with another element. Oxygen is a tasteless, odorless, colorless gas with a strong tendency to unite with other elements to form oxides. It is the most abundant element in nature, furnishing nearly half of the total composition of the earth's crust. Twenty-one percent of the air is oxygen. It is so much a part of the earth that everywhere man digs, he finds oxides or compounds of oxygen. Its most striking characteristic is its tendency to combine with all other known elements, except flourine, bromine and five or six others which are very rare. It readily combines with metals, the rusting of iron being the result of oxidation—iron rust is iron oxide.

Oxygen has a particularly strong tendency to combine with carbon and hydrogen for which it has a tremendous *chemical affinity* or attraction. It combines with hydrogen to form water, with carbon to form carbon-dioxide and carbon-monoxide. Oxidation may take place slowly or rapidly. Rapid oxidation is a process known as burning. Fuels are composed largely of carbon with which oxygen combines rapidly, giving off heat. Even iron will burn in pure oxygen, if first heated to red heat before being plunged into the oxygen. The rusting of iron, which takes place in the open air, is an example of a slow process of oxidation.

As everybody is familiar with burning, or rapid oxidation, let us use this phenomenon to make clear what takes place in foods when they are oxidized. Oxygen unites with different substances most readily at different temperature. Apply a lighted match to a piece of paper and it ignites readily and burns quickly. If the same lighted match is applied to a stick of wood or a piece of coal, it will fail to ignite these. Oxygen is distributed loosely among the tiny fibers of the paper and the paper is completely surrounded by oxygen in the air, hence it quickly ignites; the wood and coal are more compact than paper and must be heated to a higher degree before they will ignite. Coal requires a higher temperature than wood before it will catch fire.

The temperature at which a substance will ignite is called its *kindling temperature*. Slow oxidation of substances may take place at a comparatively low temperature and oxidation is always going on in practically all substances around us, being increased or decreased with any increase or decrease of temperature. It is more rapid when things are hot, less rapid when they are cold. The important fact that I want to stress at this point is that: *as the temperature of any substance is raised the tendency to unite with oxygen is increased.*

Applying what we have just said to foods, oxidation of foods takes place more rapidly at a high temperature, as in cooking, and more slowly at lower temperatures. Foods also oxidize at room temperature, but, as in the rusting of iron, this is a slow process. Foods have been defined as oxidizable substances. When they have been oxidized they are no longer serviceable as food. This is to say, the more oxidation has taken place in a food the less food value it has.

It is necessary to point out that the more intimately any substance comes in contact with oxygen, the more readily does it combine with this element. Nature protects the vital structures of plants and animals from oxidation by surrounding them with structures—skins, barks, etc.—that do not readily oxidize and that prevent the oxygen of the air from coming in contact with their inner structures. So long as the skin or bark is unbroken, the internal structures of the plants and animals are protected from immediate contact with the oxygen of the air and do not undergo oxidation. Once this protecting envelope has been broken and the oxygen comes in contact with the inner structures, there is a strong tendency for such unions to occur. A break in the skin of an animal is followed by bleeding and the formation of a tough, hard scab that seals out the oxygen. A similar thing occurs in plants; there is a flow of sap which hardens and protects the cut.

Fruits and vegetables are surrounded with a tough outer capsule or skin that is designed as an effective barrier against oxidation. But when this is broken, or the fruits and vegetables are cut or peeled, this permits oxygen to reach their inner and now unprotected structures, so that, they begin immediately to oxidize, consequently to lose food value. When we peel an apple and slice it so that we admit the oxygen of the air to its inner structure, it soon turns brown. This same thing happens when we peel and slice a peach or banana. This browning of the slices is due to oxidation. Such foods will oxidize at ordinary room temperature, but they will oxidize faster at a higher temperature, as that used in cooking.

When foods are sliced, diced, cut, hashed, shredded, or otherwise broken into small bits, and their inner structures are subjected to contact with the air, they undergo oxidation. The finer they are grated or sliced, the thinner the slices, the more of their inner structures come into contact with oxygen, hence the more oxidation they undergo. The longer these sliced, cut and shredded foods are permitted to stand before they are eaten, the more oxidation they undergo.

Nuts that are ground in making nut butters, milk that is sprayed in the process of drying (dehydration), juices that are extracted from fruits and vegetables, are all permitted to come in contact with oxygen and undergo more or less oxidation in the process. It will be noticed that in nature milk flows directly from the producer to the consumer without coming in contact with the air. In this state, the milk has an entirely different flavor than it has after it has been in contact with the air for some time. The same thing is true of all other substances that come into contact with the air. Apples and peaches do not only become brown from contact with air, they also taste differently after such contact. Nut butters do not taste like nuts. Foods lose both food value and palatability from oxidation.

When fresh fruits and vegetables are chopped into small pieces, or when tomatoes are sliced thin, there is rapid oxidation of vitamin C. For example, when lettuce is shredded it loses eighty per cent of its vitamin C in one minute. The loss is almost as rapid in tomatoes when these are sliced thin. The same thing is true of the vitamin C in oranges, cabbages and other fruits and vegetables. Ripe tomatoes seem to lose vitamin C less rapidly than do the green ones when they are sliced. In all green leafy vegetables, the destruction of vitamin C by oxidation, when these are chopped or shredded, is marked. The mere act of grating raw apples or raw potatoes causes a complete loss of vitamin C. Comparable losses of other vitamins have also been shown to occur when foods are thus sliced, cut, shredded, grated, etc. Thus it will be seen that one may buy vitamin rich foods and then prepare them in such ways as to lose most of their vitamins.

The reader should see the significance of these facts and readily see that the grating of salads is destructive of food value. The present wide-spread use of machines that cut fruits and vegetables into fine particles and liquify them, is a distinct evil. The wide-spread practice of making fruit and vegetable juices and drinking these also permits of great losses of food values. The patient fills up on great quantities of juices to get plenty of vitamins, only to have his vitamins destroyed by oxidation.

It will always be best to take our foods whole, or, if they must be cut, cut them in large pieces. Tomatoes may always be served whole instead of slicing them. A head of lettuce may be cut in half, but it should certainly not be cut into small pieces or shredded. Cabbage may be cut in large pieces. There will be some loss, even, in this way, but the loss will be insignificant when compared with the loss that occurs when cabbage is shredded. At the *Health School* we have, throughout the entire length of its existence, served our salads whole. There has never been any grating, dicing, shredding, etc., practiced.

Much of the damage done to food by cooking is due to oxidation—heat being the catalytic agent in this instance. It was early discovered that the application of heat to foods destroys vitamins. Even comparatively low temperatures, such as that used in pasteurizing milk, are enough to destroy many of the vitamins of foods. How much of the vitamin content of a food is destroyed by cooking depends upon:

1.—The method of cooking employed.
2.—The temperature to which the food is subjected.
3.—How long the food is cooked.
4.—How much the food is cut up before being put on or in the stove for cooking.

Cooking destroys in part, if not wholly, the oxidizable factors of foods. This simply means that cooking "burns" those portions of foods that the body ordinarily oxidizes. Once these substances have been oxidized, they cannot again be oxidized in the body, hence they are useless as food. Heat, by speeding up oxidation, turns food into ashes before it is eaten. For example, certain of the amino acids are destroyed by the regular processes of cooking. Two very important amino acids, Lysine and Glutamine are destroyed by the cooking process. The losses that are produced by cooking may not result in serious trouble until later in life and all of their effects do not show up for two or three generations. For example, Dr. Pottenger demonstrated that cats fed pasteurized milk and cooked flesh could not reproduce after two to three generations. They usually died of arthritis, heart disease, or gastro-intestinal complications.

It is significant that when Dr. Pottenger had fed his cats on cooked foods for a few generations, they not only developed many very serious defects, including, finally, loss of the ability to reproduce, but they also became homosexual and lost their normal endowments of hereditary racial sex characteristics. Some day, perhaps, we may know just how much similar eating practices have to do with the growing *alikeness* of the sexes in this country. Tests have shown that with large numbers of boys and girls, it is impossible to tell them apart by their anatomical differences of height, shoulder and hip dimensions, etc. Viewed nude from the rear, they were identical in appearance. Accompanying this wiping out of distinguishing sexual differences, there is the growing increase of sterility in both sexes. In Vol. V of *The Hygienic System*, I have shown that food is master of heredity. These recent findings serve to confirm what I have shown there.

The loss of minerals from foods in the process of cooking is of three kinds, as follow:

1.—There is the leaching of minerals from the foods as these run out into the water in which they are cooked, or as they run out into the pan in the juices of the food. When foods are boiled their mineral losses are great, more so if they are cut up before boiling.

2.—There is the evaporation of some of the minerals, as, for example, the evaporation of iodine. In the process of pasteurizing milk, and in this process the temperature is relatively low, twenty per cent of the iodine content of the milk is lost by volatilization. Sulphur is lost from cabbage and onions in the process of cooking.

3.—There is the alteration of some of the salts of foods so that they are no longer usable by the body. An excellent example of this is the change that occurs in the calcium and phosphorus in milk in the process of pasteurization.

It used to be asserted by the advocates of cooking that heat bursts open the membranes or capsules that inclose the starch and other nutrients of vegetables, and thus renders them more susceptible of digestion. This was particularly thought to be so with regard to the starches of cereals, legumes and potatoes. Raw starch was thought to be almost indigestible. The researches of Strasburger and Heupke in Europe and of Hastings in America have shown this supposition to be incorrect. Indeed, the digestive juices digest the unboiled or uncooked vegetable cells as readily, or more so, as the cooked ones.

Viewed from every angle, the application of intense heat to foods constitutes a great waste of nutrients. The enzymes in foods, the roles of which in human nutrition are not yet fully understoood, are also destroyed by heat. Let us look at milk again. Pasteurizing milk destroys the following enzymes contained in the milk: *protease, lactase, diastase, lipase, salolalase, catalase, peroxidase, aldehydrase, amylase* and *phosphatase.* It greatly impairs the value of chlorophyll and spoils the iron salts in foods. Animal feeding tests indicate that the regular processes of cooking reduce the nutritional value of food by at least one-third, thus lending strength to the statement that we are nourished by the uncooked and but partially cooked portions of our foods and made sick by the thoroughly cooked portions.

By now it should be evident that the chefs and the mistresses of the kitchen cannot be trusted with our physiological welfare. These turn our a never ending array of heterogenous mixtures that tax the strongest digestions; cook our foods until they have lost the greater part of their food value, salt them, pepper them, spice them, sweeten them, put vinegar or other such material on them to hide their insipid character and feed them to us as the finest selections from among their many choice recipes. The alien taste given to the foods by the mixings and seasonings make the adaptation of digestive juices to the digestive requirements of the foods impossible, while the near foods, tars, charcoal and ashes that constitute a great part of these abominable concoctions of the kitchen are materials that should never be taken into the human stomach.

Salt is Poisonous

CHAPTER XIII

Civilized man has become so corrupted by fraud and treachery that when he is not engaged in cheating his neighbor, he is busily engaged in cheating himself. For example, he is so in the habit of falsifying his bread with mineral alkalis—potash, sodium chloride, bicarbonate of soda, saleratus, etc.—vile adulterations that at once destroy the natural flavors of everything they touch, and occasion impairment of the stomach and nutritive apparatus as well as impairment elsewhere in the body, that he dislikes his bread without these. The practice has grown so inveterate that men and women are prone to suppose it natural, even necessary, and having confounded their original perceptions of taste by constitutional violations of its attraction, and having lost the consciousness of true health, they can really no longer tell whether they are doing right or wrong.

Sodium chloride (common table salt) is but one of many salts known to the chemist, but it is almost the only one that we have come to think we must add to our food in order to be well nourished. Epsom salt is often taken, as a cathartic (table salt may also be used for the same purpose) but we never think of it as a food. It is popularly thought of as a "medicine," never as a nutrient. In certain diseased states physicians do give certain salts, of iron, calcium, etc., as "medicines," but, as has been previously shown, this is to no avail.

Sodium chloride is not an exception to the fact stressed in a previous chapter that the body must get its nutritive elements, with the exceptions of oxygen and water, in organic form. Sodium and chlorine are both normal constitutents of the body, but they must both be taken in the form of organic salts, if they are to be used. Table salt passes through the body and out without undergoing any change. It is not metabolized as are organic salts. It never becomes a part of any of the body's tissues and is not employed in the production of any of the body's secretions. Contrary to popular opinion, its chlorine is not used in the production of hydrochloric acid in the stomach.

Being useless, salt is a poison, hence its use is a waste of life's energies. That it may be used as an emetic, or as a laxative is due to the fact that it is a poison. Bastedo, a standard author in pharmacology, materia medica and therapeutics says that, "under some circumstances" *sodium chloride* (common table salt) is poisonous. He says that in some sections of China people who commit suicide commonly do so by drinking a pint or more of a saturated solution of common salt. He also mentions cases of poisoning from intravenous injections of concentrated solutions and from the use of saline substances given by rectum. He tells of seeing an infant die from an enema of 1:16 salt solution that had been incorrectly labled "normal saline," and of gangrene in another from a salt solution used in hypodermoclysis. He refers to fatalities reported by Campbell, Brooks and others from the use of saline enemas. Finally he mentions a "salt fever" due to dehydration.

It is not, however, correct to say that salt is a poison "under some circumstances." A substance is either a poison or it is not—circumstances are not involved. Any substance, when taken into the body, is either a food or a poison. It is the one or the other depending on whether or not the body can use it; that is, whether or not, it can be transformed into tissue or used in the production of secretions.

Common table salt, *sodium chloride,* is at all times and under all circumstances, non-usable; hence, it is always and under all circumstances, a poison. That it is not always fatal is due to the fact that it is rarely taken in fatal doses. A strong salt solution is often used as an "emetic"—this is to say, it is used to induce vomiting. Thousands of people are in the habit of drinking a glass of salt water before breakfast each morning to induce bowel action. Both the vomiting and the bowel action are means of expelling the salt from the digestive tract. At the same time, there is increased heart action, so that it is said to stimulate the heart.

Salt is eliminated with difficulty when it has gotten into the bloodstream. Much of it is thrown out through the skin. Indeed most of the solid matter in sweat is sodium chloride. Heavy salt users, who perspire much, have so much salt in their sweat that it is more like brine than anything else, and when their clothes dry, there is often sufficient salt left on them to streak them with white lines and blotches. Their tears are also salty, while the tears of the non-user are not.

Sylvester Graham tells us that he was told by a Dr. James, formerly of the U. S. Army, "that in the summer of 1836, the soldiers in the remote Western frontiers used no salt with their food when he was with them, and that he found their sensible perspiration to be as free from the taste of salt as pure water." In the summer of 1948, I had occasion to walk for some distance at a fast pace and, as a consequence, perspired freely. I took a quantity of sweat from my face and tasted it. The taste was so like that of distilled water, with not the least saltiness, that I made a second test to confirm my first taste. It was the same.

Certain portions of the race have used salt so long that we have come to think of it as a normal practice and to think that man, as well as certain animals, resorts to salt eating instinctively. Nothing could be further from the truth. The alleged instinctive craving for salt that is supposed to exist in both man and many lower animals, is as mythical as the much talked of "salt licks" that animals are said to visit. Just how man first came to use salt is not known, but it seems to have been added to food after he learned to cook his foods and rob them of their organic salts. Salt was added to restore the lost flavor. Animals in the wild state never get salt, and it must have been wholly unobtainable by primitive man. As already pointed out it is wholly innutritious, a poison, and certainly not a needed addition to the diet.

It is certain that man has not always used salt. Tieresias, in the *Odessey*, speaks of men who know not the sea, "neither eat meat savoured with salt." Salt eating was first introduced into America by Europeans. The same is true in certain parts of India—the Todas, for example, being first introduced to the practice by their European conquerors. There are still parts of Central Africa where salt is a luxury confined to the rich. The Numidian nomads in the time of Sallust never ate salt, while the Bedouins of Hadramut and certain Sudanese tribes at the present day do not touch it. In a paper addressed by E. Steinbach to the Geographical Society (British) some years ago, he says that the inhabitants of the Marshall Islands, a Pacific Ocean group, never salt their food, not even with sea salt, not a grain of common salt has to this day been sold for that purpose by the dealers settled in the islands." It has not been found easy to seduce and debauch all "primitive" tribes and induce them to acquire the salt-eating habit.

Students of Thoreau will recall that he abandoned the use of salt after he made the surprising discovery that the Indians did not use it and maintained a high standard of health and physical efficiency without it. It will also be recalled by students of literature that Robinson Crusoe's Friday did not use salt. Indeed, a careful study of the history of our own European and American people will reveal that its general use is a rather modern custom.

The juices of spinach, beet tops, chard and other greens, cooked in a waterless cooker, so that no water is added, are so salty that it is difficult to believe that no salt has been added to the food. All wholesome natural foods contain an abundance of organic salts that are needed by the body and are useful. But it is useless to take these various salts in their inorganic forms. The calcium tablets, phosphorus compounds, iodine capsules, and tinctures of iron supplied by the drug stores and prescribed by physicians, are utterly useless. They are worse than useless, they are positively poisonous.

Get your salts, your minerals, from unprocessed, unrefined, natural foods—preferably from fresh raw vegetables and fresh ripe (but uncooked) fruits. White flour has been robbed of seventy-five percent of its minerals in the milling process. White rice has lost practically as much of its minerals. White sugar has no minerals left. Cooked foods have lost much of their minerals. Cooking and processing of foods robs them, not only of their substances, but of their savour. Baked apples have no appeal to our gustatory sense. We are forced to add sugar and spice to make them tasty. Not so an uncooked apple. Nature richly savours her foods and if we do not spoil them, we will find no apparent need for harmful additions in order to relish them.

Fragmentation of Foods

CHAPTER XIV

As the investigation into the chemistry of foodstuffs continues the matter becomes increasingly more complex. More and more factors are discovered and there follows at once, upon the discovery of each new factor, the effort to isolate it and to put it up in bottles and boxes so that it may be sold over the drug counter. There also follows the effort to produce it synthetically, so that the manufacturers may be independent of the normal sources of supply. The public, deriving its dietary information from the newspapers and advertising matter that reaches it, is misled into paying high prices for both types of "just as good" (perhaps better) substitutes for whole foods.

We have become so accustomed to the practice of dividing foodstuffs into their various nutritive factors—proteins, carbohydrates, fats, minerals, vitamins, etc.—that we often miss the importance of the whole food. Indeed, we have long since ceased to talk of foods and have learned to talk of proteins, or of calcium, or of vitamins. When we undertake to compare one food with another, we talk of the relative proportions of protein, or of essential amino acids or of vitamin B_1 in each food. We think of a food as superior merely because it possesses more protein or a higher percentage of whatever vitamin may be, at the time, in the headlines. Thus we learn to place values on the various foods according to piece-meal evaluation and lose sight of the whole food.

Nature does not turn out proteins, but whole foods. Her vitamins are integral parts of a complex whole: her minerals are not isolated food factors, but parts of the whole. In plain English, we do not eat calcium, but lettuce; we do not eat protein, but pecans; we do not eat sugar, but dates. This is the normal way of eating and no substitute that has yet been offered equals nature's plan of eating.

There is an interdependence among the various elements of the diet that has become obscured by this fragmentation of foods. The reciprocal relationship between interacting elements determines the use and value of these. Let us look at protein. Having completely lost the idea of whole food as this is produced in nature, we have come to place higher or lower values on particular parts of foods. Thus it is, that, we have been led to believe that muscle meat is the best source of protein. But, in this, we miss the fact that, in itself, muscle meat is a very inadequate food. Much depends on the proper balance and constitution of proteins and other complex and indispensable substances, for the manufacture of which the plant alone possesses the secret. It is not protein, *per se,* nor carbohydrate, *per se,* nor vitamin B complex, *per se,* but due proportions of all the requisite elements of nutrition, in order to meet, in the most efficient manner, the total needs of the developing infant and functioning adult organism, that is required if good nutrition is to be guaranteed.

The present-day diet of Americans is very largely denatured. It is made up of white bread, white rice, demineralized corn meal and other denatured cereal products, pasteurized milk, white sugar, sulphured dried fruits, sulphured syrups, canned fruits and vegetables, cakes and pies, and of thoroughly cooked foods. Although, such a diet cannot be made adequate by the addition of vitamin extracts and synthetic vitamins, nor by the addition of minerals from the drug store, the professed aim of the present promoters of such food fragments is to enable people to continue eating their denatured foods and supplement these with the fragments and still be properly nourished. It is a commercial program that seeks substitutes for foods rather than tells the people the truth about their diet.

The present attempt to build up a balanced diet by separating parts of foods from their nutritional associates and rearranging them according to arbitrary standards, none of which are accurate, is but a commercial program which the people have been misled into accepting and even to regarding as superior to nature's own nutritional program. We go even further than this, we decide that there is a deficiency of some particular food factor and we greatly overfeed on this factor, in total disregard of the two well known facts, that: 1.—There are no isolated deficiencies (deficiencies are always multiple and in the very nature of things, cannot be otherwise); and 2.—No use can be made of isolated food elements; all food elements are assimilated in association with other food elements and to over-feed on one, without, at the same time, supplying due proportions of the associated elements, is to waste the factor that is overfed.

Beginning in the latter part of the last century with the emphasis on phosphorus, which the millers added to flour, after they had taken out the organic phosphorus compounds of the wheat in the process of making flour, we have had emphasized and fed to us in pellet and powder form, such food constitutents (some of them drugs, others of them fragments of what were once foods) as, calcium, iodine, flourine, vitamin C, vitamin D, vitamin B₁, vitamin B complex, wheat germ, rice polishings, sea weeds, dried, powdered and compressed alfalfa, powdered skimmed milk, fish-liver oils, shark-liver oil, amino acids, chlorophyll, black strap molasses, gluten bread, bran, yogurt, etc., etc. One-by-one these have enjoyed a brief heyday of popular-ity, as one-by-one they were exploited by the dietitians, pseudo-dietitians and physicians. If, just now, the greatest emphasis is placed on proteins, this is because, having made the complete circuit and not having anything new, just at present, to exploit, they are forced to begin all over again. Once they determined food values by burning the foods and measuring the amount of heat they pro-duced in the process—*caloric value*. At present, they discuss the *biological value* of the proteins in the food. None of these things are valid means of measuring the total value of any food.

Today few food factors have not been separated from their partners in natural foods and packaged for sale at fancy prices. Liver extract, given hypodermically rather than through the digest-ive tract, cod-liver oil, gelatin, vitamin extracts, synthetic vitamins, mineral concentrates, amino acids, (natural and synthetic), chloro-phyll (both extracted and synthetic), powdered skimmed milk, milk sugar, and other fragments of foods, represent the present approach of the so-called scientific world to the problems of nutrition. The millions of living examples of the failure of this program, together with the many thousands who have died because the program is a fallacy, should be sufficient to convince the most skeptical that this approach to the nutritional problems of man is radically false.

Sugar was among the first food factors extracted from their natural sources and eaten by those who dislike natural foods. The more sugar is extracted, this is to say, the more of the original food is removed and the more the sugar is "purified," the less value it possesses and the more harm results from its use. The proper way to eat sugar is to eat the whole sugar-containing food. Eat dates, figs, grapes, raisins, bananas, etc. What is true of sugar is equally true of all other food factors. Powdered skimmed milk is rich in protein, but it has lost much of its value in the process of separating the cream from the milk and in the drying and powdering processes. When amino acids are removed from the foods in which they are naturally contained, they are separated from their nutritional partners, and like sugar, the more they are purified, the less value they possess.

The fact that some of the isolated food factors now sold are derived from plants does not mean that they are the equal of those contained in the plants, themselves. The processes involved in extracting them from their plant sources reduce their value. It will always be best to eat whole plant foods rather than isolated fragments of plants. Let us not be overawed by the pretentions of egotistical chemists that they know better how to prepare our foods than does nature. All too many chemists suffer with a self-destructive egomania.

This effort to feed man upon food fragments resembles in many ways the old drug system that we are trying so hard to get away from. Not only are the fragments put up as pills, powders, and in liquid form to be taken in doses of certain sizes and frequencies, but they are also, very commonly given by hypodermic injection. There is altogether too much effort being made today to by-pass the human digestive tract and feed through the skin. Too many needles are being pushed through the covering of the human body and too many substances sent into the blood stream in this manner. Nature's whole scheme of human nutrition is being neglected for commercial reasons.

Perhaps we should not be surprised to find medical men resorting to such false "feeding" practices, but when the formerly drugless schools of so-called healing resort to this plan in ever growing proportions, it should cause us to stop and ask: *are we not being shunted down a dangerous blind alley?* One may associate with naturopaths but a short time before he learns that the great majority of them are most interested in what they term "injectibles." They actually prefer to give synthetic vitamins by injection, to giving vitamin extracts orally. They have taken nature out of naturopathy. To a growing extent this is also true of osteopaths and chiropractors.

Reading the advertising material issued by the manufacturers of food substitutes, one may well imagine he is among a group of old line homeopaths, for they talk so much of "potencies," as well as of dosages that they sound like the homeopathic physician. No one would guess from their talk that they are supposed to be talking of food factors. But it does not take long to understand that what they mean is that it is all right for you to eat white bread, provided only that you swallow daily, a certain number of "potencies" of their vitamins; that white rice is a good food if you swallow two capsules a day of "sixteen-in-one" mineral concentrate, etc.

The manufacture and sale of such products are also justified on the ground that our soils are so depleted that the foods grown on them are inadequate. They are such poor foods, at their best, that, they must be supplemented with minerals and vitamins from other sources. Without desiring to minimize the importance of soil, without desiring to imply that much of our soil is not badly denatured, I would point out that the evils of our poor soils are being grossly exaggerated by those who peddle food supplements. They find this to be good advertising for their wares—it is their chief sales talk. Glib-tongued salesmen and writers of advertising copy talk so much about the poverty of our soils, the evils of commercial fertilizers and the dangers of spraying of fruits and vegetables that, they have great numbers of people afraid to eat fruits and vegetables. They have them believing, not only that these foods are poisonous, but also, that they are so poor that they contain little or no nourishment. While there is a basis of truth in what they say, their exaggerations are designed to sell concentrates, extracts, synthetics, etc.

Manufacturers of "food supplements" stress the fact that the great majority of Americans suffer from varying degrees of malnutrition, ranging all the way from border-line states to marked degrees of malnutrition, and assume that this is all due to the fact that they are eating inadequate foods. They assure us that these inadequacies can be made good by eating their "supplements."

Malnutrition, it should be emphasized, is the complex effect of many antecedents. But the manufacturers of "supplements" ignore this fact and say that, since it is impossible for everybody to grow his own food, it is best to obtain the missing food factors by taking "food supplements." The food factor turned out by the manufacturer, often parading as a scientist specializing in nutrition, may be any particular fragment of food that it be may thought possible to sell at tremendous profits.

But is should ever be borne in mind that isolated food factors do not possess the value of the same factors in normal association with the other food factors contained in foods. Nature puts up her foods in complete ensembles and our efforts to separate the various food elements and put them up in bottles and boxes have not been very successful. Science is better at building bridges than at building men. In this latter, we must follow the ancient, the primeval pattern.

It is obvious to the student of this matter, if he carefully observes all of the "food supplements" manufactured, and reads the claims made for each, that the poor victim of inadequate foods must purchase a great variety of food supplements and use these daily. He needs iron and calcium and iodine and other minerals; he must have B_1, B_{12}, D, X, Y, Z; he must have various amino acids; he must have chlorophyll, etc., etc., and he must have a different "supplement" to supply each of these needs. The program becomes expensive and, if these "foods" are injected through the skin, also painful.

What Jean Bullitt Darlington calls the *"synthetic or compensatory* school of nutrition" is made up of those men and women, commonly regarded as authorities in the field of nutrition, who, to use Mrs. Darlington's words, "belittle the importance of the natural vitamin or other nutrient, obtained in the natural way in the proportion provided by nature," in her own food products and who "promote this artificial, compensatory type of nutrition," for commercial reasons. All essential nutrients can be had from natural foods and dangers are inherent in the commercial program that substitutes extracted and synthetic vitamins, minerals and other food essentials for natural foods. Manufactured concentrates, whether of vitamins or minerals, or amino acids, or sugars, or fats, sold by commercial interests who are determined, at all costs, to maintain the unsound position that *substitute* and *compensatory* substances are just as good (probably better) as nature's own products, cannot possibly provide for superior nutrition for those who eat these substances.

We have one group of food processers—the millers, rice polishers, manufacturers of "breakfast" cereals, the dairymen, etc.—busily engaged in robbing natural foods of essential nutrients and selling half-foods, and near foods to the public. We have another group of food processers—the manufacturers of "health" foods and of vitamin preparations and mineral concentrates—busily extracting from other sources and packaging for sale to the same public, the elements and vitamins of which the first group rob the staple articles of food. Neither group is willing that the people shall have natural foods without the processing, for in the sale of the processed foods lies the source of their huge profits. The dairy industry and those physicians and nutrition ex-spurts who hang on to the financial teat of the dairy industry, tell the public that the loss of vitamin C in milk from pasteurizing is of slight consequence because it can be compensated for by a few spoonfuls of orange juice or tomato juice. They ignore, in this statement, the obvious fact that this adds to the cost of feeding children and is prohibitive to many families; that many mothers know nothing of the substitution value of juices; that pasteurizing damages milk in several important particulars for which no amount of juice will compensate; and, finally, that the unaltered natural product is always better than altered foods plus substitutes.

This same unintelligent program is followed with wheat. First all of the vitamins in the wheat and seventy-five percent of its minerals are extracted and discarded in the process of making white flour. Then, the manufacturers of substitutes sell the people wheat germ, "vitamins" and mineral concentrates with which to supplement their white flour. Calcium preparations are especially emphasized in this matter. The same elimination of minerals and vitamins takes place in making white rice; then, the people are sold rice polishings, synthetic vitamins and mineral concentrates with which to supplement their white rice diet.

As a great part of the diet of the present-day American is processed in this way, either at the processing plant, the canning factory, or by the cook in the kitchen, supplements to the diet are offered for every purpose. In the days when phosphorus was regarded as the most important element in the brain and nervous system and it was declared "no phosphorus, no thought," the millers actually added inorganic phosphorus compounds to white flour after they had removed most of the phosphorus from the wheat in milling.

If we can learn to eat natural foods without processing them and without destroying them in the kitchen, there can be no apparent need for these *compensating substitutes* for food. The "supplements" and "reinforcers" may all be relegated to that *Limbo* reserved for the commercial products that have had their day and have passed to make room for other such products.

Food elements must be used together. It is very true, for example, that at least a half dozen, perhaps more, food factors are involved in the intricate process of producing a hard tissue such as tooth enamel. Phosphorus is just as important as calcium and neither is usable in the absence of the other or in the absence of vitamins C and D. Neither are the vitamins of use in the absence of the calcium and phosphorus.

The process of building tooth enamel is no isolated process. It is not done in the teeth. It is done by the body and almost every function of the entire body is involved in the process. Digestion of food is as much a part of tooth building as it is of muscle building. The work of the heart in circulating the blood or of the lungs in supplying oxygen is part of the process of tooth building. Hence tooth building is related to the integrity of the whole organism. Not the nutrition of the teeth alone, but of the body as a whole, determines the kind of teeth we build.

This is the reason the spectacular results of taking vitamin B_1, for example, that we often read about, is just a lot of super-heated air. This is the reason vitamin extracts and concentrates, mineral concentrates and other types of food extracts have little value. This is also the reason that nutritive deficiency is never singular. It is always deficiencies that are produced by any food inadequacy.

Unless the ensemble of the diet eaten meets the ensemble of the needs of the body, the body suffers. Feeding excesses of one element or another never corrects the deficiencies in the conventional diets of our country and time. Liebig well stated this principle in his *Law of the Minimum* in these words:

"The development of living beings is regulated by the supply of whichever element is least bountifully supplied."

We can use one element of our food only in proportion to the supply of other and related elements. We can build with one element only so much structure as we have supplies of other elements also needed in the structure. We can produce secretions with one element only in proportion to the amounts with which we are supplied with other elements needed in the secretion. Here are a few important facts I want to impress upon my readers:

We do not yet know how much of any food element the body needs.

We do not yet know all of the elements that are structural and functional constituents of the human body.

We do not know that all of the vitamins have been discovered.

We do not know that there are no other and hitherto unsuspected food factors in foods that are as essential as those that are known.

These things being so, there can be only one safe source of nutriment, only one source that is capable of supplying us with all the known and unknown food elements. This source is natural foods.

In fresh fruits and green vegetables and nuts, or the juices of these, are all the minerals and vitamins and high-grade proteins, and other substances needed by the growing, developing human body to bring it to a state of physical, mental and moral perfection and to maintain it in this state indefinitely.

Fresh foods; green foods; whole, natural foods; unprocessed, unrefined foods; foods that have not lost their substances nor had their vital values deteriorated by heating, drying, cooking, canning, and refining processes are full of the elements of superior nutrition. Someday, we hope, at least, this simple fact will be recognized by our people.

What this country needs is a great teacher, one who, with the eyes of a superior being, can see the roots of our troubles, the causes of man's perennial lassitude, constant seeking after stimulants, the causes of his deterioration, weakness, decrepitude, impotence and suffering; one who possesses a deep knowledge of the secrets of nature, who knows the almost magic virtues of fruits, raw vegetables and nuts; and who can stir our sleeping people as no man ever stirred them before.

Piles of shattered pottery, superfluous stewpans, crushed baking ovens, and the ash-heaps left from the burning of "food" factories, refineries, etc., would be found in the wake of such a savior of our nation. Our people must be made drunk with enthusiasm and wild with eagerness for a new life based on a new and superior nutrition. The man who can stir this nation to its roots and bring it back to a state of pristine health and perfection will be greater than he who builds an army, greater than a scientist or inventor who devotes his talents and energies to perfecting some new engine of destruction.

Deficiencies

CHAPTER XV

Deficiency is a lack. It means that there is something missing. A *deficiency disease* is one "due to lack of essential constituents in the diet, such as vitamins;" or, it is one "due to defective metabolism." Chief among the "deficiency diseases" are scurvy, pellagra, berri-beri (multiple neuritis), osteoporosis and osteomalacia, keratomalacia (softening of the cornea), anemia and tuberculosis. Many other diseases are also attributed, in whole or in part, to deficiency.

Most of our knowledge of "deficiency diseases" is based upon animal experimentation. In these experiments a dietary deficiency is deliberately created and there is a strong tendency to regard the results of these experiments as final. In other words, there is the assumption that, since a "deficiency disease" can be produced by a deficient diet, then all "deficiency diseases" are the results of dietary deficiencies. I shall here take the opposite view: namely, that "deficiency diseases" are rarely due to deficient diets, but that they are, in most instances, due to defective metabolism.

In taking this position, I do not want to be understood as saying that there are no famines, or that on ship or in jail, or shipwrecked at sea one may not be inadequately fed, nor do I deny the evils of the predominately denatured diet nearly universally eaten in this country. I do not assert that deficiency may not result from dietary inadequacy in famines, or under exceptional circumstances in those who consume too little natural foods, but I do deny that this accounts for more than a small percentage of the cases of deficiency that abound. At the same time, I think that the border line deficiency that exists in our people who are fed on a predominantly denatured diet is the groundwork for many troubles not ordinarily regarded as "deficiencies."

Certainly there is iron deficiency in anemia, but this does not mean, at least in the great majority of cases, that there is not sufficient iron in the diet of the patient to supply the iron-needs of the body. On the contrary, in most cases, there is an actual surplus of iron in the diet. In pernicious anemia an excess of iron-containing pigment is found in all the viscera. Hunter even found that in fatal cases a large amount of iron—driven out of the circulation—was contained in the spleen. This reveals that there is more than enough iron in the body of the anemic patient to provide iron for his blood, but that it is not being utilized.

Another proof that anemia is not due to a lack of iron in the diet is seen in the fact that the anemia improves on a fast, which certainly supplies no iron to the body. There will be a marked increase in the number of red cells during a comparatively short fast. This shows that there is a store of iron in the body, but that, for some reason, it is not being used. The evidence shows that the iron in the food and that stored in the tissues is not being appropriated; that assimilation has failed. This is defective metabolism. What we witness in these cases is not a lack of iron in the diet, but a failure to utilize iron. The deficiency is not of dietary origin.

It is customary to give iron in these cases. The failure of the program is attested on all hands. Indeed, the failure is so obvious and has been so for so many decades that we marvel that it was not abandoned long ago. The iron supplied is usually some preparation of iron from the drug store and this is, as previously shown, useless and harmful. But feeding food iron also fails to remedy the anemia. What is to be gained by feeding patients iron-rich foods when they already have a large supply of iron stored in their tissues of which they can make no use?

As utilization of iron is influenced by many factors—the nutritional status of the individual, the form in which the iron is taken, the presence or absence of associated food factors in the diet (for example, iron utilization is partially dependent upon the presence of calcium, also upon the presence of copper) merely feeding iron-rich foods is not sufficient to assure its utilization.

Anemia is often seen in the plethoric, the obese, the corpulent, the pursy. It is supposed to mean a deficiency of iron, but giving iron fails to remedy the trouble. Giving mineral elements in the form of drugs fails to correct the deficiency. Trying to "build up" these people on "plenty of good nourishing food" (they are already overweight and plethoric), fails to restore health. **Blood trans-**fusions also fail. Giving liver and liver extracts fail.

The improvement seen in the blood in anemia and in the bones in rickets while fasting and the effect of sunshine in preventing the development of rickets in spite of a faulty diet, show unmistakably that in a great majority of cases of deficiency, factors other than dietary inadequacies are involved. In many cases these extra-dietary factors are the sole cause, the diet being adequate. A diet may prove fully adequate under one set of circumstances and very inadequate under another set of circumstances that make a heavy demand upon the body. For example, a diet that may be adequate for the idler may be very inadequate for the heavy worker; a diet that may be adequate in the tropics may be inadequate in the far north; a diet that is adequate in summer may prove to be inadequate in winter; a diet that is adequate for a woman under ordinary circumstances may prove to be very inadequate for the same woman during pregnancy and lactation.

In anemia it is not sufficient to supply iron to the body; it is essential that the patient shall be able to appropriate and use the iron supplied. His digestive and assimilative functions being much impaired, it is not possible that he can appropriate the iron supplied until these are restored to functioning efficiency. The failure of digestion and assimilation from whatever cause is the most common cause of deficiency. This is true of both mineral and vitamin deficiencies. If we can forget chemistry for a minute and realize that the body takes an active part in the utilization of the elements supplied, we may understand that it is vitally important that it be able to take that active part when foods are supplied.

What I have said of iron applies equally to all of the minerals of foods and to all of the other factors. Failure to assimilate vitamins is much discussed by so-called "biochemists." They have devised a whole catalogue of measures to compel assimilation when they find such failure, but they completely ignore the causes of the failure of assimilation, hence they fail. In anemia, for example, there is something wrong with the digestive and assimilative functions, and if these are not restored to the point where the patient can take care of, or appropriate the iron that is in his food, he will grow progressively worse despite dosing with iron, copper and chlorophyll. The same fact is true of all the other minerals, and vitamins of food.

If a few people out of a community of well-fed, healthy looking people, living on very much the same foods from the same sources, show evidences of deficiency, while the rest of the people of the community enjoy ordinary health, there must be something else than diet in the lives of the few who show deficiency to account for the deficiency. If these few are failing to assimilate the minerals and vitamins and amino acids contained in their foods, there must be causes other than dietary to account for the failure of assimilation. These other factors that impair the nutrition of the body are ignored by the "biochemists." But it should be obvious that if they fail to assimilate the minerals and vitamins brought to them in their foods, the cause lies, not in the foods, but in their other habits of living.

It is necesary to examine these people, to determine their personal habits, individual environments, manner of cooking, their state of mind, their poised or overworked emotions, their overeating, wrong eating, lack of sleep, their working habits, etc. We must do this in order that we may discover the cause of their failure of assimilation. Worry can cause as much deficiency as wrong diet. Emotional irritations, frustrations, inner conflicts, disappointments, grief, anxiety, etc., are among the common causes of nutritional impairment. Not until we have found and corrected the causes of impairment is there a possibility of restoring normal nutrition in these patients.

Besides a correction of the habits of living, these people need physical and mental rest. They may even need physiological rest (fasting), they certainly do not need a visit from the boys of the laboratory. They do not need drugging.

Vitamin Therapy

CHAPTER XVI

Occasionally a man lectures over the air, and he seems to lecture regularly before audiences over the country, who tells his audiences of the evils of our faulty dietary. He dwells at length on the many losses to foods in the processes of manufacture and of the failure of health that flows from the use of such foods. Then, he tells his hearers that there are three ways they can overcome the evils of our civilized diet. The first of these is the impractical one of going to some South Sea Island and living like the natives. The second is to go each year and spend a few months in an institution devoted to proper feeding. The third one is the one he recommends. It is that of using a supplement to your diet made up of minerals and vitamins.

He tells his audiences that he lives in hotels as he travels over the country; that he eats the same foodless foods that they do, as he eats in hotels and restaurants; that he takes two level teaspoonfuls daily of the powder that he recommends. This powder is composed of dried plant substances of several kinds and is said to contain all of the minerals and vitamins that we need for our daily supply. The advice is: go on eating the denatured, demineralized, devitaminized, pickled, embalmed, hashed, fried, baked and boiled diet that is customary and, then, eat the two spoonfuls of mineral-rich, vitamin-rich, powdered vegetables and you will be well nourished and will attain good health and remain in good health. He emphasizes the alleged fact that health is dependent solely upon the foods with which we feed our bodies.

At no time, during the course of his whole lecture, does he hint that there is another and a saner way of supplying the body with the essential nutrients—that of eating natural or unprocessed foods. That you may get all of the vitamins and minerals you require, and to spare, from fresh fruits and fresh uncooked vegetables is a fact that he cannot afford to tell you, for if he were to do so, it would spoil his chances of selling his inferior product. The commercial world has, for years, sought for some suitable substitute for a normal mode of nutrition, one that can be sold over the drug counter at huge profits. The whole of the present program of vitamin-mineral therapy is but part of this commercial scheme.

Instead of telling the people the whole truth about their foods and about their eating practices and, also, about their many other mental and physical habits that help to produce and maintain sickness, they tell them half truths and then sell them various commercial preparations that are made to look as much like the drugs of their childhood as possible. Like commercial physicians, who advocate giving extracts of glands of animals and laboratory-synthesized imitations of the secretions of the glands of animals to the sick and invalid, instead of teaching the people to live to conserve life's powers and capacities, and thus keep the energizing glands of their own bodies secreting their own hormones, these peddlers of food extracts and synthetic imitations of foods suggest to the people that, they continue on in their sins and have the penalties remitted by swallowing the various indulgencies that they have for sale. All of this is true because we, as a people, and the professions in particular, are submerged in commercialism, and the profession and food salesmen look upon each patient as an asset—a good physician, like a good vitamin salesman, is a good business man.

The physician frankly calls his use of glandular extracts "substitution therapy;" the administrators of vitamins do not so speak of their own substitutes for the normal sources of vitamins. It is an obvious fact, however, that vitamin therapy is an effort to substitute vitamins for, not only an adequate and normal diet, but a normal or rational mode of living. When vitamins are given to a patient who suffers with arthritis and nothing is done to correct his mode of eating and living, it becomes obvious that, just as "immunizing" vaccines and serums are intended to make unclean living safe, so vitamins are intended to make unphysiological and unbiological living safe.

There is too much of a tendency to substitute vitamins, real or imaginary, for a sane mode of life. Instead of correcting or removing the cause or causes of the patient's suffering, he is given a vitamin to take at intervals and causes are ignored. In this particular, there is very little difference between giving a vitamin pill and giving any other pill.

A man smokes heavily, drinks freely, uses coffee and other caffeine-containing drinks daily, over eats, eats a diet of denatured foods, eats haphazardly and indiscriminately, worries a lot, gets insufficient sleep, takes mineral oil for his constipation, does not get any exercise or sunshine, works in a poorly ventilated office or workshop, over indulges in sex and in a variety of ways enervates himself and thus grows progressively more toxemic. The vitamin therapist is prone to ignore all of these many causes for disease and to sell the patient a box or a bottle of the latest vitamin preparation. As he probably smokes himself, he does not stop the patient from smoking; as he occasionally gets drunk, he does not warn the patient about his own drinking habits. As he uses tea and coffee and eats a lot of denatured foods, he sees no need to have the patient eat natural foods; as he is addicted to most of the bad mental and physical habits of the patient, he ignores all of these and sells the poor victim of ignorance and misinformation a bottle of high-priced pills. Vitamin therapy is but one more of the profession's millions of efforts to *cure* disease without removing cause.

I know a vitamin salesman, representative of a manufacturing firm, who attends the meetings and conventions of the naturopaths here in the state of Texas. I have no doubt that he also attends the meetings and conventions of the other schools of so-called healing. He is a heavy smoker and when he attends a convention, he brings along a liberal supply of whiskey, the "best" brand, and freely dispenses it among the naturopaths, not all of whom drink. I see his customers drinking and smoking, eating denatured foods and drinking coffee. I once sat (I did not eat) with them at a banquet. It was held in a hotel and the food consisted of the usual hotel fare—fried or broiled steak with all the "fixings," white bread, overcooked vegetables (and not much of these), coffee and pie. I saw a number of them eat two and three cuts of pie, while others of them drank from two to three cups of coffee, putting three to four cubes of white sugar in each cup. Most of them smoked. The vitamin salesmen, including the previously mentioned one, were present at the banquet. There was one woman naturopath present whose daily eating is about the same as that of the banquet. She is a chain smoker and drinks freely of strong coffee, eats only white bread and a predominately denatured diet. Daily she has her injections of "vitamins." Thin, weak, hollow eyed, black circles under eyes, sick—she laughs at any sensible advice about living. Vitamins will sooner or later make her well in spite of a mode of living that is daily producing and adding to her troubles.

Vitamins won't *cure* the effects of gluttony while the over eating is continued. Vitamins can't *cure* the effects of inebriety while the drinking continues. Vitamins can't *cure* the effects of a diet of denatured foods while these foods continue to be eaten. Vitamins can't restore potency to a sensualist while he continues to practice sensuality. Vitamins can't be made to substitute for exercise, or rest and sleep, or sunshine, or fresh air. Vitamin therapy is a fraud and a delusion.

Most of the "evidence" offered in favor of vitamin therapy is based on laboratory experiments in which animals are first fed diets that have been deprived of one particular vitamin. Only in the laboratory are deficiencies of only one food factor fed to animals and even here, in ultimate results, the resulting deficiency, is not single, but multiple. The preponderance of evidence is to the effect that all deficiency states are not only multiple, but are in varying degrees deficiencies of all the necessary minerals and vitamins, with some deficiency of other food factors.

It should never be lost sight of that no human being ever lives the life of the laboratory animal and that in real life no scurvy is ever remedied with *ascorbic acid,* no pellagra is ever remedied with *nicotinicmide,* no anemia is ever remedied with *iron* and no beriberi is ever remedied with *thiamine.* Any piecemeal approach to dietary inadequacy is as deficient as the average diet. Optimum nutrition requires, not only an over-all adequacy of the diet eaten, but an over-all adjustment of all of the non-dietary factors of nutrition. Man's ills are not to be remedied by fragments, but by proper use of all of the related elements of his basic needs in *organic unity.*

It is often stated that in marked deficiencies it is necessary to feed vitamins in quantities greater than they can be obtained from food stuffs. Even if this were true, and it is an unproved assumption, it would not justify feeding such excesses of vitamins to those who are not suffering from such gross deficiencies. In all deficiencies it is essential to feed whole foods, not isolated food factors, for the reason that there are no isolated deficiencies; also for the reason that vitamins are valueless in a vacuum. They are useful only in connection with their associated food factors—minerals, amino-acids, sugar, fatty acids. Feeding large quantities of vitamins and not supplying proportionate amounts of the other food factors, wastes the vitamins.

The statement that optimum nutrition could be obtained from natural, unprocessed, non-synthetic foods except for the fact that we are not "big" enough eaters to get enough vitamins and minerals into our systems from food alone is commercially motivated. That nature's own plan of human nutrition is such a complete failure as this statement indicates is not a matter to be seriously considered. The manufacturers and sellers of vitamins—natural and synthetic—promote this idea in the interest, not of your health, but of their profits. There is no need for supplements to a normal diet.

It has been shown repeatedly that the ability of the body to utilize vitamins from different sources varies greatly. For example, babies can utilize vitamin A from the carotene of carrots or spinach in ten times as great amount as they can get it from a similar dosage (in terms of *international units*) of the various fish-liver oils now sold to gullible mothers. Indeed there are ample grounds for believing that all vitamins as well as all minerals, fats and proteins are more easily secured from vegetable than from animal sources.

Fresh, uncooked fruits, nuts and vegetables will supply the body with a super-abundance of the known and unknown vitamins, all the minerals, studied and unstudied, with fine sugars, easily digested fats, and proteins of the highest grade as well as with any other unknown food-factor that may be discovered in the future.

The controversy that now rages between the advocates of natural vitamins and the advocates of synthetic vitamins should leave us cold. Both sides to the controversy refer to commercial products and not to the vitamins in foods. Even those who straddle the issue and think that natural vitamins are superior in some instances and synthetic vitamins are superior in others refer to the pills and extracts and not to vitamins in foodstuffs. Those who would feed you natural vitamins would feed you pills made of vegetables, first dried and then ground to a fine powder and then compressed into a pill, or they would feed you oil taken from the livers of shark, cod and other water animals. All of these products are inferior as sources of vitamins to natural, unprocessed foods.

It is thought that in the natural B complex there are elements that are as yet unknown and have not been isolated. Some of them are supposed to be present in very minute but important amounts—in "micro" amounts. Their nutritional significance may be very great, but it is impossible to include them in any synthetic product that may be produced in our present state of ignorance.

For the informed individual there is no question about which is best, synthetic or natural vitamins. The synthetic products are not vitamins and are even poor imitations. What is more, they lack the trace elements and other minerals that are always associated with vitamins in nature. Bear in mind, also, that no complete analysis of foodstuffs and no complete analysis of the human body has ever been made. It is not yet possible to tell, by chemical means, what is and what is not needed in foods. Nature puts up the required elements in her food products and we are well adapted to secure our needed nutrients from her sources. When we eat her products we do not miss the trace elements and other associated elements that are always lacking in the synthetic products.

In a lecture delivered in Canada a few years ago, Edward Mellanby, of England, stated that "improved dietary habits in Canada, especially in the rising generation, would result in better mental and physical health, the disappearance of much sickness and physical disability, and a great reduction in the need for doctors and hospitals." Perhaps it is the realization of this fact that prevents physicians and doctors of all schools from becoming seriously interested in dietetics and in the improvement of the nutrition of the people. This may account for their continued adherence to commercial preparations in their feeding of infants and patients. Particularly do they delight in talking about vitamins instead of teaching the people to eat adequate diets.

"Super-Foods"

CHAPTER XVII

The Devil builds chapels wherever God erects a house of prayer, and, as Defoe has it, "it will be found, upon examination, the Devil has the largest congregation." This is strangely true in the realm of diet. It is not only true that the great majority of people eat and prefer the common denatured and inferior foodstuffs that are everywhere eaten, but it is also true that, when some of them break away from the conventional diet and make an attempt to find a more wholesome mode of eating, the majority of them are misled by the claims made for the superiority of the many substitutes for natural foods that are now offered the public by manufacturers and salesmen.

One of my correspondents once very seriously urged me to give more attention, in the *Hygienic Review* to such "high pressure vital foods" as cod-liver oil, brewer's yeast, wheat germ, blackstrap molasses, and yogurt. Today certain of these foods, among which is powdered skim milk, are now frequently referred to as "wonder foods." Honey and apple cider vinegar are also included by some among the "wonder foods." The many exaggerated claims made for the healing virtues of these foods are made by those whose motives are purely commercial.

Like synthetic vitamins and mineral concentrates, they are offered to the public as supplements to their diet of white sugar, white bread, white rice, denatured cereals, canned vegetables, sulphured fruits, embalmed meats, pasteurized milk, candy, cake, pie, etc. Instead of teaching the people the truth about their diet and trying to lead them into rational eating practices, they offer them "supplements," so that their diet of foodless foods may be rendered adequate. There are diet compounds, also, that are said to "contain all the minerals for the body in organic form," which are offered to the people as a substitute for a much needed dietary revolution.

There is also a search for long-life foods and the people are being led to believe that they can prolong their lives by eating freely of high grade proteins, brewer's yeast, powdered skimmed milk, yogurt, black strap molasses, honey, vinegar, etc. The modern Ponce de Leons search, not for a magic spring, the waters of which restore and prolong youth, but for foods that have this magic power. This search is of a piece with the ancient search for an *elixir vitae* that would enable man to live for hundreds of years, if not forever. It is the same as the search for the Fountain of Youth. As soon as men give up the effort to discover special chemical compounds, or a special pool that will guarantee them long life in spite of every possible reason why they should die young, they turn to something else in their age-long quest for some holy grail. Gland extracts, gland transplantations, rays of various kinds and foods, have been looked to as sources of length of life. Perhaps Metchnikoff started this food way to long life when he popularized the sour milk fad. He asserted that it was responsible for the long life-span of the Bulgarians, who actually take but little sour milk and are not a long lived people.

Not until the present frenzied search for food specifics and food panaceas has run itself out can we hope for sanity in the approach to food and feeding. Food is now the new magic—it is the mysterious compound that will do what we once expected drugs to do. Foods now *cure* without the necessity of removing cause; they now prevent, also without the necessity of avoiding cause. They are replacing drugs and serums in the armamentarium of the magician. This absurd eulogizing of special articles of food in each case, being greatly altered products, and imputing to them peculiar virtues, is, when not a purely commercial trick, the expression of childish credulity.

One of these peddlers of "wonder foods" urges proteins and more proteins—emphasizing, with the exception of yeast, only animal proteins: meat, egg, milk, cheese. He stresses the fact that powdered skim milk is a rich source of protein and points out that besides being a rich source of protein, yeast also contains seventeen vitamins. He also stresses the richness in minerals and vitamins of blackstrap molasses. But, with all the vitamins contained in these foods, he urges fortifying the diet with vitamin extracts taken daily. He urges vitamins and more vitamins. His scheme of feeding is to get a redundancy of amino acids, vitamins and minerals, it seems not to matter what kind of minerals, into the body. Take the proteins and vitamins in great quantities, even if you do not need them. As nature made no provision for us to get adequate vitamin D, he advises fish-liver oil in capsules.

The idea is rapidly gaining ground that, if a thing is good, we must over-eat of it. We must have a super-abundance of this or that vitamin, or of this or that amino-acid, or of this or that mineral in order to get enough. The evils of redundancy are being completely ignored by the new school of overfeeding. Today, they dose their patients with special foods or special food factors as the medicos dose theirs with drugs, and for the same reason. They are not feeding people to nourish them but to *cure* them. Foods are no longer nutritive substances, but *medicines*. They are *elixirs* of one kind or another.

Your gum-willies, who write and talk about diet, have decided that all human ailments are the results of deficiencies. To prevent them, to remedy them, we need only provide ourselves with a super-abundance of the vitamins, minerals or amino-acids that are deficient and, presto! we can live longer and look younger. They have created a fool's paradise in which they sport themselves for a brief time and then pass to that bourne from which no man returns.

That life is more than food and the body more than raiment, that man shall not live by bread alone, is a principle that these men never heard of. That living is more than eating, that we cannot eat ourselves into the millenium, that we need something in life other than the B complex and amino-acids—these are matters that these men seem incapable of thinking about. In their works they talk only of foods and they write about their foods as a De Kruif might write about an anti-biotic.

These miscalled dietitians offer the people only altered and denatured food products. Not only this, but one of them actually declares that natural foods are dangerous and unusable. One man declares that salads are harmful to many people, acid fruits are harmful to many more, spinach robs the body of lime, coffee stimulates the adrenals and is needed by many people, sunbaths are harmful to many more. He finds that at least seventy-percent of people are harmed by salads. Of course, if nature's products are hurtful, we must depend on the manufacturers for their "superior" products.

Honey, which is a poor food and much inferior to sweet fruits as a source of sugar, is urged upon the gullible public as a miracle food. Yogurt, which is an inferior form of sour milk (having been pasteurized and boiled before culturing), is another "superior-food," that is sold at big profits. Cider vinegar, the poisonous product of fermentation of apple juice, is urged in certain quarters as a superior source of food values.

A large part of the nutritional problems of both the North and the South grow out of our refusal to eat natural foods. Our preference for the manufactured articles—those that have been demineralized, devitaminized, denatured, standardized, pasteurized, homogenized, cooked, canned, frozen, and in other ways rendered less valuable as foods—creates dietary problems that are not adequately solved by the present reliance upon supplements and substitutes. We go to great lengths to spoil our foods and then complain about the climate. We live on a diet of white flour products, degerminated and demineralized corn meal, denatured cereals ("breakfast foods" that stick to your ribs), white sugar, pasteurized milk, embalmed flesh foods, canned fruits and vegetables, candies, cakes, pies, etc., and expect to render such diets adequate by "supplementing" them with fish oils, brewer's yeast, wheat germ, black strap molasses, honey, yogurt, powdered skimmed milk, cider vinegar, etc.

If we purchase fresh fruits and vegetables from the stores and vegetable and fruit markets, or if we take these from our own gardens and orchards, we refuse to eat them until they have been cooked out of all resemblance to food. Spinach is cooked until it is black and mushy and no one is able to tell from its taste, what it was before cooking; cabbage is boiled until it is unrecognizable; potatoes are peeled, boiled and mashed, apples are baked and then drowned in sugar (white sugar), peaches are stewed and plenty of white sugar added, nuts are roasted, perhaps salted. We eat so little unchanged, unspoiled foods that we can't possibly have optimum nutrition and, then, we blame our poor nutrition upon the climate. If it were not for the so obvious fact that the same kind of diets produce poor nutrition in warm climates, it might be possible to sustain such a position.

How true it is that he who fills his belly with substitutes often abolishes his hunger for real foods. The food manufacturers and the physicians feed people on counterfit "foods" so that the people know not the value of the genuine article. It is like the receipt of truth—people reject truth because they are so filled with fallacy that they cannot receive truth—"there was no room at the inn" for the mother pregnant with the saviour child. Truth is often born in a manger (and all too often left there to languish) because the inn is so filled with crowds of thoughtless revelers that there is no room there for its birth.

We are offered all manners of supplementary food factors ranging all the way from supplementary roughage to supplementary vitamins, minerals, amino acids, chlorophyll, etc. Even if these things possessed all the value their manufacturers say they possess, their use would not make the conventional diet of denatured foods adequate. On the other hand, natural foods will be adequate without the addition of the supplements. It is important that we teach people how to get back to a normal mode of eating rather than that we offer them substitutes for a natural diet. The "compensatory" program is a commercial program, not a program of sane nutritional practice.

It must be emphasized that science does not yet know all of the factors essential to human nutrition, nor does it understand all of the correlations of the various food factors, so that it cannot, at least in its present state of ignorance, put together arbitrarily, a balanced system of diet.

Diet and Wellbeing

CHAPTER XVIII

Animal experimentation is often very misleading in its tendencies and results. Experiments are often of too short duration to give ultimate results; their results, at best, can apply only to the animal upon which the tests are made and are not strictly and broadly applicable to man. All too often the diets fed to the experimental animals are deliberately designed to prove what it is desired to prove—this for the reason that the "research" is subsidized.

While there is a fundamental unity in all animal life, from animalcule to man, there are specific differences, even between closely related species, that render animal experiments often very misleading. There is only one experiment that can be relied upon when we are trying to determine what diet is best for man, and this is the one that is performed upon man. A diet that proves to be best for rats or guinea pigs, is not necessarily best for man.

A pigeon can take enough morphine to kill several men and fly away as though nothing happened. Hogs can take enough prussic acid to kill many men, with no apparent harm. Rabbits grow fat on belladonna, but if we were to include this plant in the salads we feed our children, we would soon be without children. The old advice to "try it on the dog," has been dignified by the term, the "biological test." I have often wondered what the "biologists" would feed us if they ever used sewer rats as experimental animals. If they were to use buzzards in their "biological tests" they would discover that rotting flesh from a hog that had died of cholera, is good food. Dogs eat bones and digest them with ease; it is doubtful if man could "get away with" a bone diet so easily. Tobacco worms live on the leaves of the tobacco plant—you try it, *worm*.

Anything we desire to prove may be proved on the lower animals, if we only use a sufficient number of kinds of animals and vary our experiments in the proper ways. Rat-pen dietetics has not supplied us with proper solutions of human nutritional problems. It would be folly to say that animal experimentation has not supplied us with some knowledge, or that it has not provided leads that have been useful, but the tendency is to rely too much on the results of these animal tests in feeding men, women and children.

Subsidized research workers have been flooding the country with the "results" of their dietetic experiments conducted upon animals. These have invaribly shown that meat is essential to healthy development, growth and maintenance. Ages of human and animal experience, which give the lie to the results of these "tests," are discounted by the hirelings of the meat trust, and the people are told that if they do not eat animal flesh and feed it to their children many dire calamities will befall them.

There is a better way of studying the effects of a particular type of diet upon man. This is to study the people who live upon the diet, the effects of which we want to learn. A striking study of this kind is contained in a report of the anatomic and pathologic observations made in necropsies of Okinawans, by P. E. Steiner, contained in the *Archives of Pathology*, Oct. 1946.

This report covers 150 necropsies performed at a military government hospital from June 13 to July 20, 1945. Ninety-nine females and fifty-one males were examined. Forty of the persons examined were over fifty years old. Death was due to combat injuries in one hundred cases, to non-combat causes in thirty-five cases, and to a combination of these causes in 14 cases.

The "low incidence of retrogressive and degenerative changes" is described as the most striking finding. Although the first bloom of youth was lost early, senility developed late and many persons were remarkably well preserved in their late sixties. "The relative freedom from degenerative disease of the cardiovascular system (heart and blood vessels) was marked." Hardening (sclerosis) of the aorta was found in only seven bodies while the middlesized arteries usually showed only tortuosity. No complications and sequels of arterosclerosis were found. The hearts of these people were found to be well preserved and heart disease of any type was rare. Coronary occlusion was not found, while hypertrophy (enlargement) of the heart of the hypertensive type (that accompanying high blood pressure) was seen only once. "There were only three cases of heart disease of known clinical significance." Disease of the kidneys was uncommon. No case of contracted kidney was found and kidney stones were found in only two cases. Although chirrhosis (hardening) of the liver was common, little disease was found in the gallbladder and gall ducts. The major fatal diseases in those who died of non-combat causes were pneumonia, dysentery and tuberculosis.

Eight Okinawa physicians confirmed the results of these necropsies as being for the most part, consistent with their experiences in practice.

These findings are remarkable when contrasted with similar necropsies and the resulting findings, performed upon Europeans and Americans. In these peoples, degenerative diseases of the heart and arteries, of the kidneys, etc., are all too common. Kidney stones and contracted kidneys are common. Gall stones and diseases of the gall bladder and gall ducts are very common. Coronary occlusion, high blood pressure and enlargement (hypertrophy) of the heart are very common.

How account for these differences? Why are degenerative diseases so rare among the people of Okinawa, as contrasted with their prevalence among Europeans and Americans? No doubt several factors help to account for these marked differences. I give you Steiner's explanations. These take two forms, as follow:

1.—"A low tension, placid, though physically strenuous life."

2.—"A simple, predominantly vegetarian diet."

These people are not strict vegetarians. Their diet is only predominantly vegetarian. They do not consume the large quantities of flesh-foods, the great quantities of milk and other dairy products and the enormous numbers of eggs that Europeans and Americans habitually consume. Perhaps, also, they do not indulge in all the many and varied poison habits—tobacco, alcohol, coffee, etc., habits—that the white man indulges in.

I do not have the original report of Steiner's, but a short synopsis of it, as published in the *1947 Year Book of General Medicine*. In this condensed report there is no mention of any tumors or cancers found in the Okinawans in the necropsies performed. I take this to

—114—

mean that none were found. If this is so, its significance cannot be overestimated. It would indicate that cancer is rare or non-existent among these people.

These post mortem findings agree well with the findings of McCarrison among the Hunzas and Siks of India. They agree, too, with the findings among the animals in nature. The wide-spread incidence of cancer among carnivores and its almost entire absence among the fruitarian and vegetarian animals, the common occurence of arteriosclerosis among carnivores and its infrequency among plant-feeders, the extremely common occurrence of tumors in our protein-stuffed poultry—these and many other facts of a similar nature, all point to the great superiority of a plant-food diet over that of the carnivore, or even over that of the mixed diet. Not only are animal proteins unsuitable for nutrition (they are not even well suited to the nutritive needs of carnivores), but the flesh eater is almost sure to consume proteins in excess.

There is every reason to believe that, despite our boasted increased length of life, which is a mere statistical illusion, the general state of man's health, when compared with that of the past, has greatly deteriorated. While there are many causes for this decline in physical and mental wellbeing, evidenced by the increasing decay of our teeth, the ever mounting incidence of cancer, the progressive increase in the incidence of diabetes, Bright's disease, diseases of the heart and arteries, diseases of the brain and nervous system, etc., and the growing incidence of cancer and heart disease in the young, there can be no doubt that our wholly unnatural and very defective diet is one of the chief factors in our physical and mental decay.

The New Diet

CHAPTER XIX

This is a day of extracts and synthetics. White flour, wheat bran, sugar (cane sugar—white or brown—beet sugar, maple sugar), gelatin, glucose, and many other substances in general use are extracts. Then there are vitamin extracts, chlorophyll extracts, amino acid extracts, mineral extracts and other extracts that are substituted for foods. We are being rapidly convinced that we are no longer able to eat natural foods and derive adequate nourishment from these; we must supplement foods with various extracts.

Not content with this fragmentation of our foods, the chemists have moved heaven and earth in their efforts to synthesize food factors for us. They have produced synthetic sugar (saccharine), synthetic vitamins, synthetic chlorophyll, synthetic amino acids, etc. Most of these synthetics are made from coal tar products. All of them are toxic, none of them are useful, but the egomania of the chemist, that leads him to believe that he can usurp the place of the plant in the synthesis of food substances, has not yet spent itself. We are destined to have offered to us by the laboratories many other synthetic "foods."

I picked up an issue of a "health" magazine and I found one full page ad by a "health food" store in which were listed for use by the "health food" addict, the following substances: lecithin granules, soybean lecithin capsules, bone meal tablets (two kinds), garlic capsules, enzymes, wheat germ oil, vitamins A and D combination, Four-B formula, vitamin A capsules, Iodine ration (kelp) tablets, vitamin B-12 tablets, rose hips tablets, brewer's yeast tablets, brewer's powder, bone meal powder, amino acid tablets, wheat germ oil capsules, choline capsules, dessicated liver tablets, chlorophyll tablets, garlic-parsley tablets, vitamin A tablets, mate tea (this contains caffeine), salt-free seasoning, alfalfa tea.

This is the legitimate result of the modern effort to fragmentize our foods. We no longer eat whole foods, but extracts of foods. We no longer take them as foods, but in pills and capsules. The only whole food offered in this full-page ad is sunflower seed. We are trying, vainly, to analyze natural foods into their many and varied food factors and re-synthesize them by mixing together these fragments of foods in varying proportions and combinations, instead of eating the whole foods as old mother Nature turns them out.

One New York laboratory advertises in this same issue of this magazine that it offers the health seeker the world's finest rose hips, the "richest natural source of vitamin C." It explains that this is now "available in easy-to-take tablets." They say that they searched the world for the very richest varieties of wild rose hips and that the ones they offer "actually tested over 300% stronger in vitamin C than rose hips now available commercially from U.S. sources." They also say that their rose hips tablets are "a wonderful surprise for those who have difficulty with citrus juices." It will be recalled that not so long ago a concerted effort was made to discredit citrus juices on the ground that they destroy the teeth. sterilize males, and work other havoc in the body. Rose hips tablets are the outcome of this campaign and it is not unlikely that the producers of the various rose hips preparations financed the campaign against the citrus fruits. Although there are other sources of vitamin C in regular use in America and these are derived fresh from our gardens (pepper being one of these—I do not mean the piquant peppers), so that one does not have to search the world for wild rose hips, the commercial vendors of "health foods" are not emphasizing these fresh sources of vitamins. On the contrary, the "health food" business, as it is operated today, is determined to lead men and women as far away from natural foods as possible and to load them down with extracts and synthetics of all kinds.

As it was originally organized, the health food business was designed to supply the health seeker and the intelligent and informed individual with unprocessed foods that could not be had through the regular channels of trade. Sun dried fruits instead of sulphured fruits, whole wheat flour instead of that famous extract, white flour, unsulphured molasses instead of molasses that had been treated with sulphur dioxide, pure honey instead of the adulterated and artificial honeys that were once so freely sold, untreated nuts, raw nut butter, etc., constituted the chief stock-in-trade of the health food stores. The world's first health food store, established by the *Hygienists* of Boston (1836), sold fresh fruits and vegetables raised on virgin soils and on organically fertilized soils, without the addition of animal manures.

Those were the days when the emphasis was placed on whole foods, pure foods, unadulterated foods, unrefined foods, unpreserved foods, fresh foods, wholesome foods, not upon food extracts put up in pill and powder form and sold in fancy bottles with fancy labels and cellophane wrappers. In those days there were no "meat substitutes," for the reason that the vegetarian of those days did not think that he needed a "meat substitute." He thought of meat as the substitute—flesh foods had, during the ages that have passed, been slowly substituted for the normal elements of the human dietary. In those days, we were going back to the original and turning away from the substitute.

Today the "health food" store is the victim of the commercial manufacturing houses and the *phoney* "health lecturers" who have convinced great numbers of people that their very lives depend on swallowing a lot of vitamin pills, mineral concentrates, wheat germ oil, blackstrap molasses (burnt), powdered skimmed milk, brewer's yeast and other inferior foods and near foods.

Let me give you a formula for a meal. To a half teacup of warm water add the contents of one vitamin A capsule, two iodine ration tablets, one vitamin B-12 tablet, three rose hips tablets, three tablets of brewer's yeast, one oz. of bone meal, the contents of three capsules of soybean lecithin, three tablets of amino acids, the contents of one capsule of wheat germ, contents of two choline capsules, four tablets of dessicated liver, two tablets of chlorophyll, one garlic tablet, one tablet of enzymes containing ox gall, papain, pancreatin and duodenal extract. Stir until all of these are throughly dissolved and then eat. If not palatable, add three tablespoonfuls of white sugar, thicken with a little white flour and add sufficient agar for bulk. Obviously this formula will have to be varied, a different formula taken at each meal, else the diet will be inadequate.

Whole dried (dessicated) liver is recommended as an excellent source of copper and iron, besides the vitamins and amino acids it contains. Then there is whey for intestinal health and bone meal for calcium and phosphorus, plus iron, copper, manganese, zinc, iodine and other trace elements. Dried alfalfa leaves, powdered and put up in pill form, are expensive and not nearly so nutritious as fresh green leaves of spinach, celery, lettuce, etc., but think of the fun you will have swallowing your favorite pills. Why bother to eat foods anymore, you can always get pills and capsules. Why go to the trouble to secrete your own digestive enzymes when you can purchase enzymes from the drug store and health food store? The physician can supply you with insulin, thyroxin, adrenalin, pituitary extract, gonadal hormones, etc., so that there is really no longer any necessity for you to secrete your own hormones. Indeed, you may profitably have your ductless glands removed. The commercial houses and their handmaidens, the "scientists," have turned nature inside out and upside down and only old fogies bother to eat foods and to secrete enzymes and hormones.

Today you can get brewer's yeast, bone meal and raw liver (not one of which you should ever take into your body) all combined in one tablet. All in one tablet, too, you can get vitamins A and D from fish liver oil, vitamin B complex from yeast, vitamin B-12 (natural) dessicated liver, iodine from Pacific coast kelp, calcium, phosphorus and trace minerals from bone meal, vitamin E from vegetable oils, red bone marrow, iron and imported wild rose hips. Think of all of this in one tablet! Three tablets are a meal. Why bother to eat such out-moded substances as cabbage, okra, apples, oranges, nuts etc.? The laboratory boys have prepared for you wholesome and delicious repasts, such as no cook in her wildest dreams ever hoped to spread before you, and they are in such convenient forms that you can carry them in your vest pocket. There is no longer any need for dining rooms, tables, and dishes. We may also dispense with dish washing, while crunching a bone-meal pill from the rear leg of a chlorophyll-fed sheep. Who wants to return to paradise? Do we not have something infinitely superior?

Sanity About Foods

CHAPTER XX

It is necessary to emphasize the fact that nutritive deficiencies in the body do not always (rarely in fact) mean deficiency in the diet. It is a fact, easily demonstrated, that, the intake of food may be more than adequate, both in quantity and quality, to meet the individual bodily requirements, while, at the same time, these requirements are not met. Nutritional inadequacy resulting from an inadequate diet is referred to as a *primary shortage,* while nutritional inadequacy resulting from a failure of digestion, absorption and utilization is referred to as *secondary* or *induced shortage.* We see far more examples of nutritional inadequacy resulting from *induced shortage* than we ever see resulting from *primary shortage.*

In a condition of markedly lowered alkalinity—so-called acidosis —calcium, although abundant in the diet, will not be properly utilized. Increased alkalinity of the blood increases calcium utilization. Iron is commonly abundant in the regular diets of anemic patients and, even in the tissues of these patients, although there is failure to utilize it in blood making. As I have strongly emphasized in a previous chapter, food is not nutrition, but the materials of nutrition, and when the processes of nutrition are faulty, from whatever cause or causes, utilization of nutritive materials is crippled.

In cases of vitamin D deficiency and in various intestinal diseases, absorption of calcium, however abundant in the diet, does not easily take place. Gastric indigestion may also impair iron absorption. It is true that in many mental and physical ills, mineral and vitamin adequacy in the food eaten is acompanied by insufficiency in the body. Merely to feed more minerals or more vitamins to such patients proves to be futile. To feed more, when the patient is unable to absorb and utilize the minerals and vitamins he is already taking, serves only to add more burden to an already greatly impaired nutritive system. First let us restore nutritive efficiency—improve digestion and assimilation—and the patient will get adequate food from his diet; not before. There is failure of digestion in hyperacidity of the stomach. While this is more true of starch than of protein digestion, even the latter is crippled.

All this is not to be interpreted as a defense of the preponderantly denatured diet that is commonly eaten today. This diet, especially when taken in the quantities usually eaten, is to a great extent responsible for the nutritional impairment that renders digestion, absorption and utilization difficult. Obviously, the body even under the best of condition, will not be able to extract from food, nutritive elements that are not there. But when we see a patient feeding, perhaps overfeeding on wholesome, natural foods and still not being adequately nourished, we do not help the patient by feeding him still more of the same or similar foods. Neither is he helped by being given mineral concentrates and vitamin extracts. He can be helped only by removing the causes that have produced and are maintaining his nutritional impairment and giving him adequate rest to enable the body to re-establish normal secretion and excretion. Overfeeding the profoundly toxemic individual and expecting him to properly utilize the food is the height of the ridiculous. Overfeeding the profoundily enervated patient and expecting him to digest and utilize the food is to expect figs to grow on thistles.

Even in "orthodox" circles it is beginning to be realized that there has been and is too much tendency to study nutrition in terms of individual chemical factors. There has been the inclination to talk too much about calcium or iron or vitamin C or about amino acids, when we are going to eat whole foods, or we should eat whole foods. Nature puts up her food substances in balanced packages and we need to learn to eat these in such a manner and under such conditions, internal and external, as enable us to better utilize them. We eat cabbage and corn and spinach, and oranges, and apples and grapes and pecans and other such foods, not iron or phosphorus or vitamin B_1.

If the "biochemist" says that he can supply the body with needed minerals in powder and pill form, I reply that he can do nothing of the sort. He can pass his chemical substances through the body, but he can't get them utilized. What Berg says is tue: "When the requisite bases are supplied in the form of inorganic salts, they are excreted so rapidly that the organism suffers from alkaline impoverishment at the time when its need for alkalies is greatest." Then, after pointing out that the organic salts are retained and are on hand when needed, he says: "Thus whereas the effect of the bases in artificial mixtures of inorganic salts is restricted to a period of an hour or two after their ingestion, the bases in the natural nutritive salts remain effective over long periods." (There is but one reason the body eliminates inorganic salts as rapidly as possible, namely, they are unusable.).

The so-called biochemist does not even know all of the needs of the body—how, then, can he begin to supply its needs, even were his artificial mixtures usable? Only in whole, unprocessed, unchanged foods are all of the nutritive needs of the body to be found. A number of elements are found in the body in such small amounts, mere traces, that they are designated "trace elements." Among these are copper, nickle, tin, zinc, manganese, arsenic, silver, cobalt, boron, chromium, lithium, palladium, nolybdenum, rubidium, selemium, strontium, tellurium and vanadium. Of these, certain of them, such as copper and nickle, serve known purposes in the body, others, though found in the body may be serviceable and may be only foreign substances. It is not possible to say whether all of these elements are needed or not. Neither is it known how many other elements are present, in such minute quantities that they are not detectable by present methods. All that we can be sure of is this: *we can supply the body with what it requires of these trace elements and get them in ideal association with other elements, only if we take them as food.* Nature's own food products provide us with the food elements we require in the forms in which we can use them. Nothing else does.

The history of "scientific" dietetics is largely a history of "biochemic" blunders. First overemphasis was placed on proteins; then upon calories; then upon minerals; lastly upon vitamins, and now we have returned to proteins. At present, we are dealing with amino acids rather than with proteins as such. The so-called scientists have always tended to deal too much with individual chemical factors and to ignore the correlations that exist between the separate factors and which must be satisfied if good nutrition is to be provided. They have not been willing to accept nature's harmoniously blended food packages, as she presents these to us, but have fragmentized these and dealt with the isolated fragments. The result is dietetic chaos rather than a science of dietetics. The artificial blends and arbitrary feeding standards they have produced are ruinous in practice.

This absurd program has even led to a complete ignoring of the human digestive tract and a growing effort to by-pass this system. Today much and increasing effort is being made to feed human beings through the skin. Salt solutions, vitamin preparations, amino acids, glucose, chlorophyll, etc., are sent directly into the blood stream through a puncture of the skin. Rectal feeding by means of "nutritive enemata," the old standby of yesteryear, has practically given way to the new hypodermic "feeding." Rectal "feeding" was never successful and "feeding" through the skin is equally a failure. "Science," as we call this system of magic, is constantly searching for substitutes for natural products and the natural method of reproduction, so it seeks to predigest our foods and to give us food through the skin. The egomania of the "scientists" drives them into greater and greater blunders.

Here at the Southwestern Research Foundation in San Antonio, great effort was made to produce cattle by ova-transplantation. A whole staff of "scientists" and their assistants wasted months of time and large sums of money in the effort. They were successful in transplanting the fertilized ova, but the cows all aborted. Finally, the effort was abandoned. Old mother nature rejected their meddling with the reproductive function. Someday we are going to realize that nature resents all of our meddling with her processes and functions and that she rejects each and all of our substitutes for normal functions and processes. When we come to this realization, at least half of our "science" will be thrown into the waste bin. In nutrition, as in reproduction, we can hope to achieve desirable results, only if we conform to nature's own patterns and methods.

Laboratory findings, about which we hear so much, are very misleading when they are not translated into terms of food commodities. If these are translated into terms of "biochemic" preparations and into artificial processes of feeding, they can but lead to disaster. If, for example, we want to enrich the diet with added calcium, this must be done by adding calcium-rich foods to the diet and not by taking calcium preparations prepared in the laboratory, nor by eating powdered egg shells. Even ground bone, while rich in assimilable calcium, is not the best source of calcium. Above all, we must realize that it is not possible to provide adequate nutrition by "reinforcing" the diet with synthetic products resembling those known to be present in foodstuffs. The obvious failure of synthetic vitamins plus their toxic character should long ago have convinced us of this fact. The chemist's substitutes for natural foods produce only harm.

Two features about bone meal deserve our attention at this time. Bone is processed by chemicals in the process of making bone meal. The statement is made by biochemists that when phosphorus is administered in large amounts with calcium, as in bone meal, the phosphorus tends to precipitate insoluble calcium soaps in the gut, thus retarding the absorption and ultimate assimilation of calcium. While many authorities on human nutrition contend that calcium deficiency is the most common deficiency found in the diet of civilized man, they are all pretty well agreed that almost all diets provide adequate phosphorus. All of this would indicate that bone meal is not the best source of calcium for man.

Perhaps a few words about egg shells may not be out of place at this point. It is asserted that the calcium carbonate and certain trace elements contained in the egg shell are gradually released as the embryo bird evolves to form the complete skeleton structures of the bird at the time of hatching. It is asserted that at no other place in nature does this occur. These facts are supposed to indicate that egg shells are excellent sources of calcium and trace elements for man. My own observation of the results of egg shell feeding have convinced me that it is nothing more than another commercial scheme to "cure" disease without removing its cause. Food and not egg shells is the proper source of calcium for man. The powdered egg shell that is sold on the market has other substances added, such as citric acid, vitamin D, etc., to "enhance ionization and assimilation" — a good sales "angle," but poor nutritional science.

The so-called scientific world is wedded to the carnivorous practice and all of its dietetic advice is designed to induce mankind to eat more flesh, eggs and milk. A writer in the July 1954 issue of *Prevention*, in answer to the question "can you substitute beans or soy beans for meat" (flesh), replies: "Sometimes, but remember no vegetable food is as rich in all the essential amino acids as food of animal origin, so don't depend on beans day after day for protein."

This reply is asinine, in spite of the fact that it is approximately correct. Nobody depends on beans alone, day after day for protein. Nor does anybody depend on any one food on any day as the sole source of protein. The human carnivore is so blinded by his gory practices that he is incapable of understanding the simple nutritional practices that all vegetarians and fruitarians understand very well. He is not only led astray by his morbid appetites, but he is willing and anxious to mislead everyone else. He talks learnedly about amino acids (substances that are manufactured by plants and by nothing else) and reveals his ignorance of dietetics by assuming that one must derive his or her amino acids from some single source. If beans won't supply you with adequate amino acids, you are sunk. There is no other source of amino acids in your diet.

The protein frenzy has reached such a stage that it is now asserted that, "There is no chance of your getting too much protein." Conversely, it is asserted that, "There is every chance of your getting too little." After a hundred years of research, every bit of which has tended to show that a low protein diet is best, the protein frenzy has returned the flesh-eaters to the old high-protein standard of Voigt. The packing industry, the poultry industry and the dairy industry have the National Research Council by the throat with a strangle-hold.

The emphasis is being placed upon flesh foods, even hamburger meat, as a source of amino acids. It should come as no surprise to us that men who insist upon turning our food plants into saprophytes, as the organic gardeners are bent upon doing, should seek to make saprophytes, carnivores, parasites and even cannibals of us. You cannot, according to these pseudo-ex-spurts in nutrition, secure the needed amino acids from beans, macaroni, cereals and gelatin, therefore you must eat flesh, eggs and powdered milk. There is just no other source left from which to derive these precious building stones. Are these men deliberately trying to deceive their readers in the interests of certain vested interests, or are they so willingly ignorant that they are but blind leaders of the blind?

In the summer of 1954, Michael Graham, a British nutritionist, described to European "scientists" how to prepare rodents as food; he told them that, "A large rat needs 20 minutes boiling, a mouse needs 5 to 10 minutes according to size." An English gourmet in his audience said: "I have found that London mice do not taste as good as the ones I used to eat at Winchester." With the aid and approval of "nutritional science" modern European man is rapidly degenerating into a rank carnivore.

News comes from England that dried fish are being put into the prepared foods for cows in that country to supply protein. Our "scientists" having discovered that nature made many blunders, the greatest of which was that of not making all animals predatory, know that protein is protein and that it makes no difference where it comes from. The cow, normally a vegetable-eating animal, is now being fed on a carnivorous diet. No wonder Dr. Tilden predicted that "science" would crack the brain of this age. Already, although the practice of feeding fish to cows has been going on but a short time, reports of injury to babies fed on the milk from fish-fed cows have been made. Tests with milk from cows not fed animal foods have revealed that the milk from strictly vegetarian cows does not hurt these babies.

These are not facts from which our "food scientists" can learn a lesson. They are so determined that the normal feeding habits of man and animals shall be destroyed and the whole earth perverted in the interest of their pay masters—the owners of the food industry—that they close their eyes to every hurt that arises from their outrageous feeding plans. "Scientists" no longer study nature and her laws to understand her but to warp and distort her. They are still eating fruit from the forbidden tree—only they have ceased to eat the apples of knowledge of good. They are eating only the apples of the knowledge of evil. I must repeat that if mankind does not destroy its "scientists," its "scientists" will destroy mankind, and I do not limit this statement to the "atom scientists."

To date chemists have learned how to synthesize four of the amino acids. They are synthesized from coal tar products, as are the synthetic vitamins. Like the synthetic vitamins, they are nonusable. The chemist will someday recover from his egomania and realize that he cannot synthesize acceptible food substances. There is simply no shadow of a shade of a reason why anyone should think that there is need to synthesize amino acids. Every protein substance in the earth is made up of them and we need only to eat natural proteins to secure usable amino acids.

There are amino acid preparations extracted from food substances such as flesh and yeast. These are offered to the public as food supplements. Such commercial products are never as good as the products of digestion. It has been said that these amino acid extracts are no more artificial than is dried milk or powdered eggs. Let this be granted. Is dried milk a normal food substance? Are powdered eggs wholesome food substances? They are sold and used because there is money to be made out of the manufacture and sale of such products. Emphasis is placed upon the fact that the amino acids in these extracts are concentrated; at the same time they are said to be present in the "proper proportions as they occur in nature." These two contentions cancel each other out.

There is experimental and clinical evidence to support the statement that the indiscriminate supplementation of the diet with amino acid concentrates may easily result in a dietary imbalance that may result disastrously. This is true both of the "natural" amino acids and the synthetic "amino acids," but it is doubly true of the synthetic substances. In experiments with rats in which synthetic amino acids were added to the diet, the protein balance was so completely destroyed that the rats developed serious nervous conditions in a very short time.

Let us never forget that what is needed is not amino acids only, but amino acids in ideal combination with proteins, minerals and carbohydrates, and that, when this combination is lacking the amino acids are not usable. Let us eat proteins and leave it to the normal function of digestion to give us the amino acids contained in these. Why try forever to ignore the normal processes of life? We have not yet learned to improve upon them.

"Curing" With Diet

CHAPTER XXI

My readers are so far convinced that there are special diets for special "diseases," that there are specific foods for specific states of the body, that there are special foods to feed particular parts of the body, that there are diet "cures," that I continue to receive letters asking that I provide them with such diets and information about the "specific values" of special articles of diet. Other readers write me long winded criticism because I neglect to prescribe special diets for their ailments. A man will write and say: "Will you please send me a diet for arthritis;" a woman will write and say: "I am going to have my first baby, will you please send me a diet for pregnancy;" a young man writes: "What shall I eat for asthma?"

Do my readers want to be food faddists or *Hygienists?* Do they want to follow the ignorant advice of the Hausers, Braggs, Pretoriouses, Kordels, *et al*, or do they want to learn to live sanely? The absurd doctrine that "diet does it" is not and never was a part of *Hygiene.* Men who peddle vitamin pills, capsules of mixtures of mineral salts, sell powdered skimmed milk, black strap molasses, etc., are no more to be trusted to advise the people in matters of eating than are the crowd that prescribe cod-liver oil, shark-liver oil, gelatin, and "plenty of good nourishing food to keep up your strength." Men who regard diet as a *cure* are in the same boat with the crowd that give drugs to *cure.*

Sooner or later, I continue to hope, the people will learn that diet will not *cure* disease. Fasting will not *cure.* In fact, nothing that is known to man can *cure* anything. The living organism is self-healing and succeeds in restoring health by its own orderly processes, when not frustrated in its work by a lot of mental and physical bad habits. The practice of medicine, treating the sick with all kinds of methods, with diets, etc., is an abnormal practice arising out of vicious living habits of the people. These habits cause sickness by causing enervation. The unintelligent demand for relief has fertilized the soil on which has grown myriads of systems of "cure." When the people learn that sickness is as unnecessary and senseless as the *cures* are kavish or stupid, they will learn to live rightly and thus maintain health.

"They that are whole need not a physician, but they that are sick," puts the emphasis on health, on soundness, on integrity. The treatment peddlers and cure-mongers have always placed the emphasis on disease, for it is disease that provides them with fat incomes. The unceasing cry of the sick is: "give us cures and more *cures;*" and the treatment peddlers of all schools of *curing* meet this demand with a never ending succession of ephemeral wonder-working *cures*.

The *cures* don't last. Every school of so-called "healing" peddles its new *cures*. There is a constant stream of *cures* that follow each other in melancholy succession to *Limbo*. If a new *cure* is discovered (usually they are "discovered" very well) by the regular medical profession, it is announced in the public press with great furore, it is heralded to the world with a whole front-page display, a veritable storm of sensational publicity sweeps the country and it seems to those who suffer the consequences of their own folly, that, at long last, they are to be saved in their sins. At last they are going to be able to eat their cake and keep it; the great men of "medicine" have discovered a way to sober up a drunk man while he continues to drink. The *cure* does not last. A few weeks or a few years and it passes "unwept, unhonored and unsung" to the therapeutical Potter's field.

There have been many "diet cures." Many of my readers are old enough to recall the "miracle of milk." They will recollect that the country was dotted but a few years ago with institutions devoted to the "milk diet," or the "milk cure." The "grape cure," which invaded America while the War for Southern Independence was in progress, was revived but a few years ago by a "magnetic healer" from Africa, as a *cure* for cancer. It still has a certain vogue, but is waning. There was once the "candy cure" for colds, the "carrot *cure*" for tuberculosis, then the "carrot *cure*" for night blindness. There was the "blackbery *cure*" for diarrhea; for a long time there has been Lydia E. Pinkham's vegetable compound for the ills of women. The *cures* may come and the *cures* may go, but the *curing* goes on forever.

All the diet schemes yet devised by the gum willies of all schools of dietetics, whether their advocates know it or not, are merely different plans for substituting a supposedly less injurious plan of gluttony for the one that is largely responsible for the disease. Certain of the diet cures deliberately encourage gluttony. Edward Earl Puriton once described the milk diet as the "harmless practice of overeating on milk." That the people who were given the milk diet were overfed admits of no doubt; that the practice was harmless is debatable. Feeding six to eight quarts (I have seen patients take as many as thirteen quarts of milk a day) of milk daily is very much like giving the grape diet victim sixteen pounds of grapes a day. Certain of the gum willies of the present strenuously advocate over-eating of proteins. The old Salisbury meat diet was a diet of this character. Others have their victims guzzling fruit and vegetable juices in great quantities.

When a physician tells a patient who is suffering from habitual over eating that "you must eat plenty of good nourishing food to keep up your strength," he is in the same boat with a physician who would say to a drunk man: "you must drink plenty of 'good' stimulating whiskey to give you strength to walk." To advocate overeating of protein, by those who are already suffering from a life-time of protein gluttony, is as ruinous as would be the advice to the exhausted runner to "take more exercise." People who are sick from excess cannot be restored to health by added excess. They need to be taught to eat less.

Habits that enervate child or adult lessen digestive power. If food intake is not lessened by those who are enervated, digestive trouble follows. It is well known that cold feet will interfere with the digestion of food. Warmth conserves energy and helps the enervated to digest food and to establish normal bowel action. Those who eat within their digestive limitations will not have indigestion. Those who habitually overstep their limitations will be always in trouble.

There are but two reasons for giving attention to what we eat and these are both made necessary by reason of the fact that we are cut off form nature and her unchanged products. The first of these reasons is: *we must be careful to provide the body with adequate amounts of all of the nutritive elements.* The other reason is equally as simple. It is this: *we must eat under such physical, mental and physiological conditions as enhance and do not retard the digestion of the food eaten.* The first rule requires that we avoid the denatured foods and eat nature's unchanged products; the second rule requires that our foods be properly combined, that they be eaten when we are hungry and emotionally poised, when we are in a state of good health and vigor. Eating when fatigued, when worried, grieved, in pain or feverish, means eating when digestion is impaired.

Sooner or later large eaters reach the end of their toleration for excess, as shown by digestive impairment and discomfort after eating, and there is no remedy for such trouble except to limit the food intake to amounts within the digestive ability of the individual. A different diet, if it is also taken excessively, will certainly perpetuate the trouble. If digestive function is impaired and the diet eaten is in excess of the power of the individual capacity to digest, it hurts and does not help to feed the theoretically required amounts of calories, amino acids, etc. Laboratory standards are not recognized by the enfeebled organism.

When nerve energy is not equal to the demand required to keep elimination equal to tissue disintegration, toxic waste is retained, producing toxemia. When the body is persistently taxed in the endeavor to overcome or excrete stimulants (poisons) of all kinds and fermentation products of all kinds that arise in the digestive tract, energy is used up in excess producing enervation. This checks elimination and toxemia results. All kinds of symptom-complexes (diseases) become imminent. Overeating of bread and cereals, overeating in general, such combinations as bread and flesh, bread and eggs, bread and cheese, cereals with milk and sugar, cereals with milk alone, cereals with sugar alone, acids with starches, acids with proteins, fats and proteins, melons with a regular meal, jelly and bread, pies, cakes, candies, etc., result in fermentation and putrefaction of food in the digestive tract. Bread and milk, often fed to babies and children, is a ruinous combination. When this is followed by or accompanied with fruit, or with sugar, it is still worse.

People with full digestive power (this is to say, those whose secretions are normal) will protect themselves against bacteria, fungi, food excess, and even to a large extent, against wrong combinations, but the enervated and toxemic, those who have taxed their nerve energy untill they lack adequate energy with which to carry on the functions of life, will suffer from each overindulgence. Human eating should not be made into a mysterious something that requires a university education to understand. It is really simple and should be kept so. It is time we begin to laugh the gumwillies out of existence. Let us consign their *cures* to the same *Limbo* that has been reserved for all the other *cures* that pass in the night.

There is but one remedy for disease; namely, *remove the causes that are impairing health*. A diet *cure* that does not end the stimulant habit, that does not correct sensuality and excess, that does not educate the patient out of his emotional bad habits, that ignores the need for rest and sleep, for fresh air and sunshine, for exercise and pure water—such a *cure* is a *cure* on the order of penicillin and streptomycin.

At home, in the restaurants and hotels, or wherever one eats, bread, the traditional "staff of life," is fed in such gluttonous amounts that everybody overeats on this food. It is served three times a day at meal time, it is eaten between meals in one form or another. We have cultivated the habit of eating bread with almost everything we eat. All too often the other foods on the menu are served in such frugal amounts that the diner is forced to overeat on bread or leave the table hungry, or at least, with appetite unsatisfied. We not only take bread in excessive amounts but we combine it indiscriminately with all manners of foods.

We begin at their birth to educate our children into the practice of eating too much and too often. The habit is persisted in throughout school and college life. The physical as well as the mental worker eats too much. Physicians, especially specialists, are fond of telling the victims of this life-long gluttony that, diet has no effect whatever on your disease, you must always eat plenty of good nourishing food. Watching the stuffing process, as it is carried out in the hospitals and especially in the tubercular sanitariums, gives us a fairly good picture of what these men mean by eating plenty of good nourishing food." If our people could learn to eat within their digestive and assimilative powers, these specialists would be forced to close their offices and get jobs at honest work.

The tubercular patient goes to a tubercular sanitarium, where he readily falls in with the stuffing practice so vigorously cultivated in these institutions. Here he may eat and smoke, and smoke and eat without hindrance or protest. Here he may drink his fill of soda fountain slops at intervals. Here he is encouraged to eat like a harvest hand, although he is confined to bed and permitted no activity, because his disease is "tuberculosis" and nothing else matters in this "disease" except a super-abundance of "good nourishing food." Spit-cups galore are required to take care of the bronchorrhea (diarrhea of the lungs and air passages) caused by the eternal stuffing of food beyond digestive and assimilative capacity. The bowels and the kidneys are also forced to work over time to excrete the excess food that is forced into these unfortunate victims of "medical science."

Our people are drunk on food excess and the dietitians encourage them to eat more. They provide trick diets of one kind or another, designed to give them variations in their gluttony, but they never admonish the people to discontinue their gluttony. We tend to go to excess in everything we do and the gumwillies *cure* us of the effects of our excesses, not by correcting our modes of living, but by overfeeding us on special diets. The chiropractor will punch your spine; the osteopath will pull your leg; the masseur will maul and pound you; the physiotherapist will roast and freeze you or electrocute you; the psychologist will treat you to a round of "healing" suggestions; the Christian Scientist will assure you that there is no pain, no disease; the physician will poison you; the surgeon will remove your organs—and all of these *cure* mongers and treatment peddlers will urge you to eat plenty of good nourishing food—to *cure* you of the effects of your table excesses. With the obvious failure of this program (the failure is all around you) you still clamor for a "diet" that will *cure* you.

Natural Hygiene is not a system of diet, nor yet a complex of special diets, but a total way of life. It is not a compound of *cures* for disease, but a plan of living. It does not substitute foods, fasting, sunbathing, etc., for drugs, but uses these things because they are primordial requisites of life. We peddle no *cures* and recgonize none.

Fasting and Rejuvenation

CHAPTER XXII

In Public Health Reports (Vol. 67, No. 2, Feb. 1952) Anton J. Carlson, Ph.D., Professor Emeritus of Physiology, Chicago University, and his assistant F. Hoelzel, have a brief report on "Nutrition, Senescence, and Rejuvenescence" in which they suggest that "it is posisble that the striking beneficial after-effects of prolonged fasting may be due to . . . that the non-essential tissue used up in starvation (fasting) may include abnormal accumulations of some intermediary product of metabolism." This is more than a hint that fatty tissue and other less essential tissues of the body, those tissues, in other words, that are used first when food is withheld from the organism, serve as depositories in which uneliminated waste is stored to get it out of the general circulation. It also implies that when these tissues are broken down (autolysed) during a fast, these stored wastes are returned to the circulation and eliminated. This is precisely the *Hygienic* view and has been for more than a hundred years.

For the cumbersome phrase "intermediary product of metabolism" I would substitute the simple term *toxemia* which we define to mean poisoning by retained body waste. Excretion (elimination) is inhibited (checked) by whatever lowers nerve energy (whatever produces enervation) so that normal body waste is retained to accumulate in the blood and lymph. But it cannot be permitted to remain in these, else the whole organism will soon be saturated with it and death from poisoning result. The toxins are stored (deposited) in those less vital tissues of the organism in which they will do least harm. The fatty tissue is, perhaps, the first and preferred depository, as Graham thought.

Heavy metals, like bismuth, mercury (quick silver), etc., are stored in the bones. Some substances are known to be stored in the liver. Judging by what comes from the liver or through the liver in many patients while fasting, it may be that the liver stores much waste. An amazing variety of substances are sometimes thrown out by the fasting body. This is a feature of fasting that one must see to believe. It may not be difficult to grasp the fact that tumors are broken down (autolyzed) in the same manner as is fat, it should not be difficult to understand that the rest afforded the stomach and intestine by the fast enables the body to heal gastric and duodenal ulcers, or ulcers in the colon (ulcerative colitis), in the womb, etc., but some of the beneficial effects of the fast have to be seen to be believed.

Fasting, by creating a nutritional scarcity, forces the body to surrender superfluities and to excrete encumberances; eliminations which it cannot achieve in a state of surfeit. The surrender of surplus material is compatible with increasing powers and with processes of physiological and even biological readjustment. As an example, numbers of plants and animals exhibit a deep-seated physiological necessity for a reduction of surfeit and depredation as a pre-requisite to the reestablishment of sexual reproduction. Fasting by salmon, the Adelie penguin, the Alaskan fur-seal bull (Prof. J. Arthur Thomson says that many similar examples occur among animals) during the mating season are but a few of the examples of this reduction of surfeit and depredation by such animals. It will be noted that these animals are all predacious and voracious and enter the fasting period heavily encumbered with fat, which, is itself incompatible with fertility. Fasting, by dispensing with the superfluities and reestablishing normal physiolgical conditions, is perhaps essential to genetic recovery in such animals.

The effects of sudden "starvation" on previously well-nourished organisms (those that have been overfed on "rich" fare) in restoring the sexual organs and bringing back sexual reproduction, is well known to biologists, although this recovery of health and structure, as a consequence of fasting or abstemiousness, is never thought of by them as having any lesson for man. The aphis is seen to purchase rejuvenation by curbing its habit of depredation and returning to a more wholesome mode of nutrition: that is, by moderation and a legitimate fare. This move results in a return of the male and a return to the sexual mode of reproduction after several generations of parthenogenetic reproduction. The animal and plant world is replete with examples of the dis-aggregation of organisms (loss of structure) and loss of function consequent upon redundancy and wrong food and restoration of both structure and function by a return to moderation and right food, or following a fast. I need hardly emphasize the fact that the reversal of the conditions that led to the asexual state will also, if carried too far, arrest sexual development. This is merely by way of saying that fasting can be overdone.

In those cases of men and women who have been restored to sexual potency and fertility by fasting, in some instances, after several years of impotency and sterility, not all of them have been fat. Indeed, some of them have been much underweight at the outset of the fast. In these cases, even if not in the fat ones, no doubt toxemia resulting in catarrh of the generative system or in malfunction of the ovaries and testicles may be the cause of infertility and impotency. Impotency, indeed, may be due in some of the cases to nervous disease consequent upon a long standing toxemic state.

Physiological re-adjustment of a similar nature, but involving the whole organism, is indicated by Dr. Carlson and Mr. Hoelzel in their report. They say: "More than 35 years ago, the senior author found that a 5-day fast, undertaken to study hunger, produced highly beneficial physical and mental after-effects. Marked general improvement lasting at least 6 months was experienced by Hoelzel following a 26-day fast in 1913, and similar improvement was experienced in 1917 following a 15-day fast, despite the development of nutritional edema." While I have emphasized the fact that the whole organism was involved in the results of these experiments, it is not to be thought that the whole organism is not involved in every fast and in every change of fare. The ancient Jews purchased rejuvenation by abandoning the flesh pots of Egypt and subsisting for forty years on "manna"—plant food.

Prof. Carlson is one of the most outstanding physiologists of America. At the University of Chicago he has devoted considerable study to the subject of fasting. Much of his experimental studies of fasting have been made on animals but a great part of them have also been done with human beings, including football players. Several years ago Drs. Carlson and Kunde, one of his assitants, published the results of their findings of the rejuvenating effect of fasting in the *Journal of Metabolism*. Prof. Carlson's interest in the subject has not waned and it is reported that at the age of seventy-seven he takes frequent fasts of one to three days at a time. It seems that his longest fast has been seven days. His present assistant, F. Hoelzel, has had several fasts of much longer duration, one of them lasting forty days.

At the Second International Gerontological Congress held in the Jefferson Hotel, St. Louis, in Sept. 1951, Dr. Carlson read a paper on fasting (Sept. 12) in which he said that "After fasting, there is evidence of improvement in mental and physical activities." By fasting, he explained that he meant abstinence from all food except water. Both he and Hoelzel took only water during their fasts.

Working with rats, Carlson said that he had been able to demonstrate that the span of life could be prolonged by intermittent fasting. He was not sure just how this increased life-span was brought about and suggested that perhaps the fast does not actually prolong life, but that plenty of food shortens life. It is my opinion that this latter suggestion is the correct one. I do not believe that fasting lengthens life, but I am fully convinced that overeating shortens it— that, to use an old saw, most people "dig their graves with their teeth."

In certain low forms of life, on the other hand, the evidence seems to show that fasting actually prolongs life to a great age. Huxley's famous experiment with worms is a case in point. If any of my readers are unacquainted with these and similar experiments revealing the actual rejuvenating effects of fasting, they should get my book on fasting, which is volume III of *The Hygienic System* and read the story there.

Dr. Carlson thinks that there is lacking conclusive evidence that periodic fasting will increase the length of human life, or, to put it, perhaps, more accurately, prevent overeating from killing man off prematurely. It is my opinion that the "grand old man of physiology" has too narrowly confined his field of evidence. It is true that statistical studies of the longer life of fasting human beings are lacking and no control groups have been contrasted with fasting groups, but in spite of this, there is much evidence to show that intermittent fasting enables man to live longer than does continuous overeating.

We may also, legitimately, look at this matter from another point of view; namely that the rejuvenation and beneficial effects of fasting is a generalized benefit and is not confined to any one form of life. In all forms of life, including even plants, in which fasting has been tried, it has proved to be beneficial. In all animals of whatever kind in which the experiment has been made, the result has been a longer life span. It is hardly likely that a measure that is so generally beneficial should fail to benefit man also, and in the same way, even if not to the same degree. For example, as I have often said, I do not believe that fasting at intervals will ever enable any man to outlive nineteen generations of men, as did Huxley's worm, but I am sure that, as in the case of Carlson's rats, intermittent fasts will enable the faster to outlive the consistent gluttons.

In dealing with man, however, we must make due allowance for the great differences in individuals, such as are not found in the rats. A pen of healthy rats will show very little difference in constitutional strength, or in organic proportion and symmetry. An equal number of our cross bred and random bred fellow men will show so much disparity of organic composition that it will be difficult to believe that they all belong to the same species. The life potential of the rats will be about equal, that of the men will vary greatly.

Carlson pointed out, on the other hand, that the evil effects of overweight in man have long been known. He even went so far as to say that moderate underweight seems to be much better than overweight. How does overweight shorten life. He was not sure. He though that it might be due to the added strain that the overweight puts on the cells and organs. He theorized that overweight "may produce a poison for living cells." Whatever the explanation, the fact cannot be denied that overweight people do not live as long as normal or moderately underweight people. Here we are dealing, again, with averages—it is only in the mass that this is true. There are individuals who are underweight who die young and inidviduals who are much overweight who reach what we call advanced age. But, from the evidence we have, we are safe in saying that the fat person who reaches "old age" would live longer if not fat. On the other hand, there is no evidence that the thin person who dies young would live longer if overweight.

Carlson points out that 25,000,000 Americans are overweight. He thinks that there are probably more overweight individuals than underweight ones. An interesting question comes to mind here; namely, how much could we increase the average life span in this country by reducing these 25,000,000 people to normal weight? It is my thought that the average life span could be increased by three to five years by such reduction. Overweight people have more tumors, cancers, diabetes, heart disease, Bright's disease, apoplexy, and similar diseases than do underweight individuals.

At this same Congress Dr. Folke Henschen of Stockholm, Sweden presented the results of studies of the people of Sweden during the last war. These led to the finding that scanty diet reduces the incidence of hardening of the arteries and chronic inflammation of the heart muscle (myocarditis). He pointed out that in both Finland and Sweden, rigorous food restrictions were necessary during the war. Flesh, fat, eggs, starches, and sugars were scarce. Vegetables were more abundant. He says: "People grew thin, they complained about restrictions. But the common state of health has never been as good in Sweden as during that time. - The mortality decreased to a minimum, owing mainly to a very marked decrease of death from arteriosclerosis (hardening of the arteries) and myocarditis chronica (chronic inflammation of the heart muscle). Also gall stones were less frequently found at "autopsy."

After the war, he pointed out, when people could again get all they wanted of things they wanted to eat, the death rate from hardening of the arteries and chronic inflammation of the heart, rapidly rose so that it was soon higher than before the war. This, I believe, indicates that a people who are restricted for a period of time, and who have no understanding of what is going on, tend to go to great extremes in their eating when the restrictions are lifted. But I doubt that all of the health improvement seen in Sweden during the war (and a similar improvement was noted in England at the same time) was due to less food. I am of the opinion that much of it was due to the fact that there was also less tobacco and less alcohol, perhaps less tea and coffee, etc., for the people of Sweden, as of England, to indulge in. There was certainly a different kind of food eaten.

There was a very high death-rate among the former inmates of the Japanese prison camps during the first three to four years following the end of the war. I am convinced that these people were fed to death, or that they ate themselves to death. The highest death-rate was among those who ate most, whereas, those that ate moderately survived. Gross overeating, high-protein fare following prolonged periods of food restrictions, such as the prisoners underwent during the war, are ruinous.

The question is legitimate: If a period of restricted eating results in improved health and a lowering of the death rate in a whole nation and a subsequent period of the customary overeating results in an increase in disease and an increased death rate, will not a continuance of restricted eating, if not unduly restricted, maintain the improvement in health and the lowered death rate? Will not periodic fasts in those who refuse to control their eating in any other way, compel a using up of surpluses and an elimination of accumulated waste and have the same effects in man that it is seen to have in lower animals? More than thirty-five years of experience with fasting and over forty years of study of the subject, have convinced me that both these questions may properly be answered affirmatively. Indeed, I know that I have seen numerous patients recover health through the fast and live many years thereafter, who, except for the fast, would have been dead in a few weeks. In these cases there is no doubt about the prolongation of life.

It is interesting to note that on the day before the Japs attacked Pearl Harbor, Hoelzel submitted a short article dealing with "Some Factors in the Nutritional Determination of History," to *Science*. The article was published in *Science* for March 6, 1942. In this article Hoelzel says: "I am inclined to agree with Clendening that the importance of vitamins in nutrition is being grossly exaggerated. False hopes of simple solutions of nutritional problems appear to be raised by an over-emphasis on the value of vitamins. Indeed, it remains to be seen whether the use of 'enriched' foods and vitamin preparations will do much more in the long run than increase the incidence of obesity, diabetes and other disorders promoted by over-nutrition."

I fully concur with the implications of Hoelzel's statement. My readers, who have been with me for several years, will readily realize that he is saying the same thing that I have repeatedly said in my writings and lectures. The chief difference is that I have gone much further in discounting the emphasis that has been placed on vitamins by the gum-willies and have repeatedly warned of the evils of overeating that the vitamin peddlers were and are encouraging.

Hoelzel suggests that the common tendency to self-indulgence in the midst of plenty is one of the causes of national decline, whereas, seasonal variations in food supply, periodic famines, food scarcity during wars, and religious fastings "have apparently tended to avert the otherwise precipitate decline of nations or cultures" resulting from overindulgence. He suggests that in America "it is more important to guard against the insidious effects of dietetic excesses among the 'well fed' millions than to concentrate on raising the nutritional standards of the extremely poor." He adds that "so-called deficiency diseases may often be excess diseases—due to excessive intake of carbohydrates, fats and/or proteins." I can agree with this, as did Tilden and Weger in many of their published statements. Great numbers of the poor are overfed, but wrongly fed. The rest of our population, also wrongly fed, eat two to four times as much food as they need or can use. Gluttony is our first national sin.

Arteritis (inflammation of the arteries) and myocarditis (inflammation of the heart muscle) are due to a toxemic state to which overeating is a contributing cause. The experiences of the many men who have used fasting in the care of patients have shown that a period of fasting will end the inflammation of these organs. I have seen numerous cases of so-called "incurable" heart disease get well during a fast. Arterial inflammation, arterial hardening and arterial tension are also remedied or reduced by a fast. This is to say, food restriction is not only effective in preventing these diseases, but is also effective in remedying them, once they are established. In making this statement, which is fully borne out by my experience, I have the backing of Tilden, Weger, Dewey, Rabagliatti, Leif, and numerous others who have had vast experience with the fast. So far as I am aware, Dr. Carlson has had no experience with the fast in disease. He has demonstrated its rejuvenating effect and watched it prolong life, but he may never have observed the autolytic disintegration of a tumor brought about by the fast, nor the dissolution of gallstones and kidney stones during a fast. There is so much about the fast that laboratory workers never have an opportunity to observe!

What I say will be ignored by the world of science. I have no "scientific standing." The scientific snobs regard me as a "quack" and refuse to consider my observations as of value. I have probably conducted more fasts than any other man now living—these have ranged in duration from two or three days to ninety days. They have been in people of all ages of life, from early infancy to over eighty years of age, and in all kinds of conditions, from comparative good health to tuberculosis, cancer, and almost all other types of so-called disease. An experience of this kind may mean nothing to the men of "science." Some of them, at least, will listen to Dr. Carlson.

Babies Should Not Be Fed Starches
CHAPTER XXIII

Of all foods that man eats, starches need thorough chewing most. They require to be thoroughly broken up and mixed with the saliva of the mouth, the enzyme *ptyalin* of which, initiates the digestion of starch. The present wide-spread practice of feeding cereals, baked potatoes, bread and other starch foods to babies is responsible for much illness in them. Indigestion, constipation, diarrhea, colic, skin rashes, catarrhal troubles, tonsillar troubles, etc., are chief among the outgrowths of such feeding. Why? Because the baby lacks both the teeth with which to chew such foods and the ptyalin with which to initiate their digestion.

It is no answer to this to feed them soaked starches, mushes, mashed potatoes, gruels, etc. They still lack the ptyalin with which to digest these foods and at the same time, if they had such ptyalin, the eating of soaked starches would not elicit the flow of saliva. All starches, whether eaten by child or adult, should be eaten dry to insure thorough insalivation.

But babies can not chew cereals and dry starches. They have no teeth with which to masticate such foods. Not until they are twenty-four months old do they have a mouthful of teeth which will enable them to thoroughly masticate solid foods of any kind. The lack of tools with which to properly chew solid foods certainly indicates that nature has not *intended* that babies should be fed such foods.

Nature has provided milk for babies. Normally this type of food should constitute the food of the baby until its development has reached the stage that permits complete handling of other foods. This is true in the animal world, even among those species of animals that are born with a full complement of teeth. Little kittens cannot be so easily debauched in the matter of food. Until they attain a definite stage of development, they reject cheese, flesh and all other foods save their mother's milk. If mother's milk is absent they may be taught to take milk from other animals.

In all mammalian species the normal nursing period bears a definite relationship to the period of time required for the animal to attain maturity. Those animals that require longest to mature also have the longest nursing periods. Man requires longer to mature than any other animal in nature, hence his normal nursing period is longer than that of any other mammal. How long should that nursing period last? Among so-called primitives and among the so-called "backward" peoples, who have no supplies of animal milk with which to supplant mother's milk, the human nursing period ranges from three to five years and even longer. Nursing of children of nine years has been noted.

In man, as in the lower animals, there is an over-lapping of the nursing period wtih the period after weaning, when normally no milk is taken at all. That is, between the period during which the animal takes only milk and the time of weaning, there is a period during which it takes both milk and other foods. This period constitutes a period of transition from the exclusive milk diet to the diet that contains no milk at all. We may call these three periods the *milk period,* the *transition period* and the *adult feeding period.* The first belongs to the baby, the second to the small child and the third to the pre-adolescent, adolescent and adult.

All the efforts to work out feeding programs and dietaries, "based on the conclusions of modern nutritional research," as their authors say, which I have seen, have completely ignored the natural or normal order of feeding infants and children. When the chemist and laboratory worker analyzes a food and tests it on rats and demonstrates its food value or lack of value, he has accomplished no more than that. If he should say, after determining the food value of flesh or nuts, that, these should be fed to the infant from the day of birth, he would be "right" so far as his "researches" can show. But he would be wrong so far as the natural order of feeding is concerned. Not even the whelps of the lion, tiger, wolf, etc., get flesh from the day of birth. Indeed, they live upon milk exclusively for a definite period after birth before they ever take flesh food.

The anatomical and physiological development of the baby distinctly marks the beginning of the second period; thus it determines the normal diet of the baby. Until the child is equipped with teeth to chew solid food, its food should be milk; or milk and fruit juices. When it has developed a mouthful of teeth, it should begin to add solid foods to its diet. When it arrives at the stage where it should be weaned, there is no longer any need that it be given milk.

This is all contrary to the present popular dietary principles and practices. Today it is advised by those who are supposed to know, that, every child be given a quart of milk a day. At the same time the adult must have a goodly portion of milk each day. We are never to be weaned. We are to be sucklings all our lives. All of the talk about milk being the perfect food and its need throughout life is fostered by commercial interests that profit from the sale of the milk; for nobody advises that mothers continue to suckle their children until they are ninety years old. The dairy interests have made the remarkable "discovery" that cow's milk and goat's milk are the perfect foods.

There is another and very important consideration that indicates in the strongest possible manner that babies should not be fed certain types of solid food before they are two years old. The fact is that not until they reach this age do they secrete the salivary enzyme, *ptyalin,* and the pancreatic and intestinal enzymes essential to the digestion of starch. It is the worst type of folly to feed babies starch at a time when they cannot possibly digest it, even if fed dry and in proper combinations.

No baby should be fed starch foods before it is two years old. This rule should apply to all starch foods. It will be observed that nature has put no starch into milk. The carbohydrate of milk is sugar. If, towards the end of the period of infancy, there is a desire to give the baby some carbohydrate in addition to that contained in its milk, the sugars, of dates, sweet grapes, well-ripened bananas and other sweet fruits that the medical profession declares to be tabu for babies, should be given. These predigested sugars require no ptyalin for their digestion.

Of all starch foods eaten by man, cereals along with legumes, are the least fitted to the capacities of his digestive organs and are also least well-fitted to meet the nutritive needs of his body. Babies fed on such foods have indigestion, colic, diarrhea, constipation, colds, hives, tonsillar and adenoid troubles, and even more serious difficulties. They develop poor teeth and are soon making their regular visits to the dentist's for tooth-repairs.

Many mothers are well aware that their toothless infants are not equipped to chew solid foods, but they think that this difficulty may be overcome by mashing, scraping, pureeing, and straining the foods. Scraped apples, mashed potatoes, cereal mushes, purees of various kinds and stewed fruits are fed to babies in the hope that these may be digested and assimilated with ease. This is especially not true of starches, as the enzymes necessary to their digestion are lacking before the baby is two years old. It should be significant to every intelligent person that nature supplies the needed enzymes at the time she supplies the requisite teeth. The practice of mothers of forty and fifty years ago of chewing the food for the baby had more sense to it than the present feeding vogue. I do not approve of the old practice, which died out because the medical profession scared the wits out of mothers with their germ bogey, but it at least had the advantage of insalivating the starches before the baby swallowed them.

Feeding mushes, purees, scraped apples, mashed bananas or mashed potatoes and other foods that require no chewing before swallowing (even soaked cereals may be swallowed with ease without chewing) teaches the little fellow to swallow his food without chewing it. If solid foods are given to the baby at the right time, he will instinctively learn to chew his foods. The nation is full of anxious mothers who complain bitterly that they cannot get their children to chew their foods and these mothers are unaware of the fact that they have trained the children to swallow their foods without chewing them.

The exercise of a little common sense would save mothers and children a lot of trouble. Why should mothers heed the advice of physicians in feeding their babies and children? These physicians are not trained in dietetics. The medical colleges from which they graduated do not teach dietetics. The *materia medica* of the medical schools is composed of a few thousand poisons, but there is no food in it. Within recent years the synthetic vitamins have found their way into the *materia medica*, but these belong properly to the category of drugs.

Wrong feeding produces its most harmful effects during the years of growth and it is here that a complete revolution in our feeding programs is most urgent. Here, where the foundations of the future are being laid, it is important that adequate food be supplied, that it be fed in a way that it may be fully utilized and, also, that proper feeding habits are establbished. Nothing can be more important to the future of a people than that its children be given proper, natural food and that they be fed according to the natural order.

Dirty Waters For Health

CHAPTER XXIV

For ages men and women have been pilgrimaging to various watering places in many parts of the earth and drinking the waters of these places or bathing in their waters, or both, both to preserve their health and to remedy their diseases. Indeed, the watering places have been as popular, perhaps even more so, as the various temples of the gods and shrines of the saints, as places for the sick to be magically relieved of the effects of their transgressions of the laws of life. Many are the stories of almost miraculous recoveries that take place in the watering places.

There are many thousands of mineral wells, mineral springs and mineral waters throughout the world that are frequented by throngs of invalids from all parts of the world upon the advise of their physicians. Commonly there are physicians in connection with these wells and springs that supervise the bathing and drinking in the various conditions of the patients. What have we in these wells and springs? Just dirty water! These waters possess all the "healing virtues" of the water in any dirty pool. Perhaps none of them contain as much dissolved minerals as the water of the ocean, hence none of them are as *curative* as ocean water.

Analyses of mineral waters show them to contain such matters as magnesium chloride, sodium chloride, calcium chloride, potassium chloride, calcium sulphate, hydrochlorate, iron oxide, calcium carbonate, ammonia, aluminia, sulphur, gypsum, etc. These are elements of the soil—dirt—that are held in solution in the water. In plain English, these waters are dirty waters and the more of these various "earthy matters" they hold in solution, the dirtier they are. It is these various mineral salts that give to the waters of the various wells and springs their characteristic odors and flavors. It is these various inorganic, hence unusable, salts that occasion the diarrhea and diuresis that follow their use and that have led to the belief that they are beneficial. In other words, we are dealing with drugs—mineral drugs—in every one of these waters.

The owners of some of these springs and wells bottle the water from them and ship it over the country for sale to gullible people who cannot go to the watering places. Many thousands of dollars are yearly spent for these bottled waters. Other owners have learned to evaporate the water, thus leaving the salts behind, and have packaged the crystals thus left and ship these about for people to buy them and add to their own water. Then, there are a number of mineral preparations that one may purchase in the drug stores and health food stores with which to make one's own "mineral water," or "sulphur water." All of this has the same value as would a handful of dirt from your back yard dumped into your bath tub, or dissolved in the water in your drinking glass.

When, nearly a hundred years ago, the water of the Dead Sea was analyzed and found to be rich in dissolved earth—dirt—the *London Medical Times and Gazette* said: "No mineral water is so loaded with saline matters, or contains so much bromine, and it would be of great interest to try its effects in scrofulous cachexia, inveterate syphilis, rickets, diseases of the bones, chronic affections of the respiratory organs, etc." It was dirtier than all other known mineral waters hence it probably had "curative virtues" that all other known mineral waters lacked. It would be interesting to try (experiment) it in certain diseases that other mineral waters and other drugs failed to "cure."

The medical profession have taught and the people have believed that lime water, sulphur water, iron water, iodine water, magnesia water, and all kinds of earthy, alkaline and saline mineral waters (which are not fit to wash nor cook with), are excellent for drinking purposes, especially if one is an invalid. If they found a spring, the water of which was so foul the cattle would not drink it, they invested it with "curative" virtues. As absurd as is this notion, it seems to take well with the "learned profession" as well as with the unlearned people.

At one time, arsenical water was added to the list of wholesome and health-imparting waters. In the southern part of Cumberland, England, many streams of water originate among veins of arsenical cobalt, consequently their waters have arsenic in them. The waters were, perhaps still are, used by the inhabitants and it was thought that the drinking of the arsenic proved to be positively beneficial.

While the waters of these streams were healthful for man, no fish could live in them and ducks could not live if confined to the arsenical waters. When first used by both men and horses, the water produced soreness of the mouth and throat; this is evidence, to the medical mind, that arsenical water is good for man. If it produces disease, it will cure disease.

Every foul and poisonous thing which has become a "food," a "medicine," or a "beverage," has at some time or other received the endorsement of the medical profession. Alcohol and tobacco, tea and coffee, chocolate and cocoa, arsenic drinking, etc., are only convenient examples of this fact. French chemists shortly after the middle of the last century maintained that many celebrated waters actually owed their "beneficial qualities" to the arsenic contained in them.

A number of years ago, however, an American physician traveling in Europe and investigating the various watering places, stated that the French physicians who had had greatest experience with Vichy water, were the ones who thought least of it. No doubt this is true of all famous springs and wells. Those who know the most about them have the least confidence in them. From this category we must exclude the physicians who may own such a spring or well, or who have a hotel or sanitarium that exploits the waters of such places. For these will affirm their confidence in the waters, even though they have none at all. Their statements are dictated by their economic interests.

True to the inherent absurdities of the drug system, physicians cannot find water anywhere on the surface of the earth that is loaded with poisons without imagining it to be in some mysterious manner, remedial for all depraved conditions of the blood, and bones and breath. Some of the waters are so foul of taste it is difficult to swallow them, but it is imagined that their curative virtues are in proportion to their foulness. Some of them are possessed of such foul odors that it is difficult to go near the well or spring—some of them smell like rotten eggs—but this is regarded as an evidence of their "healing virtue."

So, today, as in ancient times, people frequent these watering places to be *cured* of their rheumatism, arthritis, gout, kidney troubles, neuritis, paralysis, "syphilis," gonorrhea, etc., etc. Faith in the "curative" powers of these various dirty waters is very ancient and very firmly fixed in the minds of most people. Indeed, this faith dates back to pre-historic times. It will not be esay to eradicate such deep-seated faith.

Sixty and a hundred years ago, when the country was dotted with numerous "water cure" or "hydropathic" institutions, it was common for the proprietors of these places to locate their bathing places near some well or spring and, in their advertising, emphasize the peculiar medicinal virtues of their water. Their packs, fomentations, wet sheets, dripping sheets, douches, sitz baths, sprays, etc., had more "curative" power, due to the presence of the dissolved soil in the water. It was the old drug conception of the curative power of poisons carried over into the "water cure." Unfortunately, as Dr. Trall asserted, the hydropathists got their philosophy from the drug system and merely substituted water for drugs. They consequently, favored drugged waters.

Dr. J. G. Webster, writing in the *Herald of Health,* July, 1863, says that most of the Water Cures, both in this country and in Europe, use either "mineral water," "medicated water," or drugs, or all three in the treatment of their patients. Priessnitz had not employed any of these but his followers soon departed from his practice and leaned towards the medical systems of the day. (This fact probably grew out of the fact that most of his followers were medical men from the various medical systems.) The heads of these watering places, says Webster, regarded these mineral waters, medicated waters and drugs as necessary to the "cure" of many bad cases. In both this country and in Europe, he says, a great proportion of the "water-cures" were located in the vicinity of mineral springs, the waters of which were lauded very highly as possessing "peculiar virtues." Some of them even went so far as to claim that their particular water was more *curative* than the waters used by other hydropathists.

Water is legitimately used in or on the human body as a drink and to cleanse it, as in washing or bathing. For both of those purposes, the purest water is best. Indeed washing the hands and bathing the body in hard waters—mineral laden waters—hardens and injuries the skin. Such water does not cleanse readily; it does not cleanse the skin any better than it cleanses the hair. It is not best for washing clothes. How foolish to think that bathing in such water is preferable to bathing in pure water! How unhygienic to drink dirty water! The drugged waters of our cities—our chlorine cock-tails, etc.—are also unhealthful.

Is there any more reason to think that impure water is *curative* than there is to think that impure air or impure foods are *curative?* If we employ mineral waters in the treatment of the sick, why not also adulterated foods and foul air? I am aware that there are those who have gas chambers into which they have their patients go to breathe various gasses—this is to say, they treat their patients with foul air—but the evidence for the value of such treatment is no better than is the evidence for the value of adulterants in foods. For health we want and must have pure water, pure air and pure food.

The time to drink is when one is thirsty and when this time arrives, there is nothing to equal a glass of pure, clear, sparkling, cool, water. Nobody has ever been able to imitate the flavor of water nor to provide even a temporary substitute for it. It would seem that the more advanced portions of the human race should out-grow the ancient superstition that dirty, foul tasting waters possess *curative* "properties" when taken internally or when applied external-ly, as in taking a bath.

Both the philosophy and the practice of the *Hygienic System* are predicated on the primary premise that things which are con-stitutionally adapted to the preservation of health, are also the proper agents with which to restore health. It rejects from its "materia medica" all poisons, animal, vegetable or mineral—all things which, if present in the body, are incompatible with the normal play of all the functions of life and which are destructive to living tissue.

Is Your Boon My Bane?

CHAPTER XXV

The old fallacy that "what is one man's meat (food) is another man's poison" has served and misled people so long and is, today, so often repeated, even by men who should know better, that I deem it wise to say a few words in combatting it.

I once saw a man to whom water was a poison. He drank a glass of coca-cola about every thirty minutes during the day to satisfy his thirst. The caffeine in this slop did not hurt him. In fact, he explained to me, that by his athletic activities he "burned up" the caffeine. But he was afraid of plain water. I have never yet met a person to whom air is a poison, but have met several who were "poisoned" by fresh air. Fresh air gave them colds, or headaches, or other trouble; foul air agreed with them perfectly.

While most people seem to agree that "what is one man's food is another man's poison," they continue to eat as though this is not true. In all parts of the country, the diets of the people are fairly uniform. One goes into a hotel or a restaurant and finds the same foods on the menus and, if he watches the great throngs of people who eat in these public eating places, he soon discovers that they all eat about alike. If he goes to the grocery stores, meat and fish markets and to the fruit and vegetable stands, he is soon struck by the fact that the housewives are all buying about the same articles of foods in total disregard of the *fact* that what is one man's food is supposed to be another man's poison. If he goes into the homes of the people and observes the foods served on their dining tables, he soon comes to realize that there is a marked sameness in the diets of the people of any community. Occasionally he will discover a person who is "allergic" to strawberries, but he never finds one who is allergic to flesh foods. "One man's meat is another man's poison," is a fallacy that is used to defend the conventional eating practices, and especially is used to defend the continuance of carnivorous habits, and to supply us with a "reason" for not revolutionizing our diet.

In mass feeding programs an even greater uniformity of diet is noted. Just as a farmer will feed a hundred hogs on the same corn, a dairyman feed the same grain and hay to his whole herd of cows and the rancher feed the same hay and grain to his horses, so, in an orphanage or a boarding school a hundred children will be served the same cereal with pasteurized milk and white sugar for breakfast; in the prisons the men will file by the kitchen with their platters and all be served the same foods; in the army and navy, large numbers of men and women will be fed the same chow, or the men will all be issued the same "K rations." All of this will be done with no thought that one man's boon is another man's bane. There is a monotonous sameness in the diets fed in the hospitals and there is no thought that the food of one is the poison of another.

The eating practices of most people are matters of habit and custom, rather than of intelligent planning. Our people are influenced more in their eating by advertising than they are by any knowledge of foods. They eat what has been made to "taste good," rather than what is truly good. They eat foods which they know contain poisons—chemical preservatives, coal tar dyes, artificial flavorings, etc.—with no thought of these poisons, and reject good foods only because they have not learned to eat them. Seasonings, rather than the flavors of foods, determine what is *liked* by their undiscriminating tastes.

Indeed, it is only when somebody suggests that intelligence and our vast store of accumulated food-knowledge be made use of in feeding ourselves and our young, that anybody ever remembers that what is food for one is poison for another. Physicians and pseudo-dietitians are especially likely to profess to believe that the vegetarian diet, though food for the few, is poison for the many. They take the position that flesh and white bread are food for everyone, while apples and celery may be poison for many. They'll tell you all of this while sucking the fool's end of a cigarette.

For the most part, the assertion that what is food for one is poison for another is applied to those articles of food that are derived directly or indirectly from the soil. Even here, it is not asserted that calcium is food for one and poison for another, or that carbohydrates are food for one and poison for another. I have never seen it stated that vitamin C nourishes one man and poisons a second.

The contention is not made against the food factors or food elements as such, but against the food products that contain these elements. And yet, such foods never enter the body of any one. Cabbage does not circulate in the blood stream. Potatoes are not rolled through the arteries and veins like marbles. Imagine a fish-eater having little fish swimming around in his blood stream! *Foods are broken down in the processes of digestion into a few uniform and acceptable substances and these alone enter the blood stream.*

"But we are not all constituted alike" protests our wise man. It may be true that life is as chaotic as this implies, but, if it is, physiologists have not found any evidence of it. Each of us starts life as a fertilized ovum and follows in the course of our evolution the same lines of development. We arrive at maturity with the same number of muscles in our bodies. We possess the same glands and have the same digestive and excretory systems.

Each of us secretes saliva containing ptyalin; each of us secretes gastric juice containing pepsin. The liver of each of us turns out bile, while the pancreas of each one produces pancreatic juice with the same enzymes. The glands of the intestines of each of us turn out the same juice containing the same enzymes.

Structurally and functionally our digestive systems are so much alike that the physiologist can't find that different constitution we hear so much about. At the same time we all require the same food factors to nourish our bodies. Everything points to the suggestion that we are constituted upon the same principles, are constructed alike, have the same nutritive needs and are equipped to digest and utilize the same kinds and classes of food substances.

I have never seen a man whose constitution was that of a dog, or that of a cow. They have all possessed human constitutions and so far as human observation can go, they are all subject to the same laws. Did anyone ever proclaim that cows, for example, are so differently constituted that some cows need and must have grasses and herbs and others cannot use these, but must eat flesh? Or, has anyone ever declared that, whereas most lions live on flesh, blood and bones, some lions are so differently constituted that flesh is their poison and they must graze like the ox?

All this nonsense about different constitutions is prated by people who haven't the slightest idea about what is meant by *constitution*. By constitution is meant the composition of the body. It is, in other words, the *tout ensemble* of organs and functions that constitute an organism. Man's constitution differs from that of the horse or the wolf, but not from that of another man.

Man is in subjection to natural law. Every organ and every function in his body renders unceasing obedience to natural law. His whole organism is constituted according to and upon immutable law. Will it be claimed that the laws that govern one man's structures and functions differ from those that govern the structures and functions of another man? Are all men subject to the law of gravity? Then all men are subject, and in the same degree, to all other natural laws.

The laws of nature are such that everything we do or fail to do either conforms to law or runs counter to it. There is no neutral ground. It is ridiculous to say that the laws of nature require one kind of practice in one man and another and opposite kind of practice in another. Habits and circumstances that are precisely adapted to the laws of life in one man are habits and practices that are precisely adapted to these same laws in another man.

Because of this false doctrine that there are many kinds of human constitutions, requiring different habits and circumstances to conform to the laws of life, we are misled into all kinds of errors. "Tobacco does not harm my constitution," says one, while another confidently asserts that "coffee agrees with my constitution." Another possesses a constitution that requires large quantities of food, while another is so constituted that he requires very little sleep. There is hardly an injurious practice and indulgence in the whole long catalogue of man's abuses of himself, that is not defended by those who practice them, or indulge, on the ground that it agrees with their particular and peculiar constitution. None of them, so far as I have been able to ascertain, have ever found that jumping from the top of the Empire State Building agrees with their constitution. But if life is as chaotic as they seem to think, there seems to be no reason why some constitutions should not be found that would need and require such jumps.

The reigning theories about allergy may seem to lend credence to the idea that the boon of one is the bane of another, but we should ever bear in mind that *allergy* is a pathological condition, rather than a constitutional difference. The *allergic* individual finds that he can eat the foods to which he is "allergic" as soon as he is restored to a

—154—

state of good health. On the other hand, I think it quite probable that the fact that large numbers of people prove to be "allergic" to a particular article of diet, such as eggs or shrimp, is at least partial evidence that such a "food" is best omitted from the diet of everyone and not merely from the diet of the "allergic" individual. Widespread "allergy" to a particular food probably indicates its unfitness for human nutrition.

Life being what it is and natural laws being what they are, what is really and permanently best for one is best for all; and what is injurious for one, is so for all.

None of the above is to be interpreted to mean that human needs do not vary under different conditions and circumstances of life. No one would be foolish enough to declare that the three days old infant and the fifty years old man have identical needs; or that the needs of man in the tropics and his needs in frigid regions are identical. Nor are the needs of the sick and those of the healthy identical. This is not due to any change in the law, but to change in conditions.

There are individual weaknesses and differences in resistance that call for temporary modifications of any program of living, but it is essential that the modification comply with the laws of life. All programs or parts of programs that violate these laws are ultimately ruinous. Variations within the law are legitimate. No variations that step outside the law are ever permissible.

Variety, the Spice of Gluttony

CHAPTER XXVI

It is a matter of common experience that we tend to eat much more food when we eat two or more foods than when we take but one at a meal. If we are eating but one vegetable we eat just so much and we are satisfied; but if we are eating two vegetables we tend to eat as much of each as we would of a single vegetable, if we have only the one or the other at a meal. For example, if we are eating carrots and have consumed all we want of these, we can go back for a serving of asparagus or spinach and apparently start eating all over again. This common experience does not prove that we need a variety of foods to supply our demands at the time; but that *a variety of foods tend to induce overeating*.

This is only one of the reasons why the common habit of eating desserts at the end of a meal is an unwholesome practice. We can always eat a piece of cake, or pie, or a dish of ice cream, or other dessert, even after we have consumed so much of other foods that we experience a sense of uncomfortable fullness. The greater the variety of foods we take at a meal, the more we are likely to eat. If we have six foods in our menus we are likely to eat much more than if we have only three. We are a nation of gluttons and much of our overeating is due to the great variety of foods that are placed on our tables at each meal. This practice stimulates the appetite and the gustatory sense to the utmost at each meal.

Indeed, it is the custom to serve the foods in a regularly graduated scale of gustatory relish. Starting with the food that gives least enjoyment and gradually working up to the food that gives the greatest relish, we end by eating two, or three or four times as much food as we actually require and more food than we would take, except for this *stimulation* of our appetites.

Having eaten all he wants of one food, the eater turns to another and still another, until he has eaten several foods. Having eaten all he needs or much more, he takes, as a final part of his meal, the article he relishes most. After eating two or three times the quantity of food he requires, he can still "top off" his meal with a piece of pie or cake or some other dessert.

It is the rule that our people continue to eat in this manner until appetite is so depraved and diseased that it becomes an imperious master. This is especially true of those on the conventional diet of *stimulating* foods. They establish a nervous "craving" for *stimulation* which is referred to the stomach for satisfaction and is in every way like the "craving" of the drunkard for his alcohol or of the morphine addict for his morphine.

A morbid appetite, thus established, which is, in reality, nothing but a morbid longing of enervated nerves for their accustomed *stimulus,* which they receive by means of food, is not satisfied when the body has received sufficient food to meet its needs, but is satisfied only when the nervous system has received enough *stimulation* to bring it up to its ordinary tone. When this stage has been reached it is all but impossible to avoid overeating. One is now a food addict and one's appetite is a despotic, even painful master. One has a powerful and painful craving or longing of an outraged and diseased nervous system, not for food, but for the accustomed *stimulant.*

Normal hunger and appetite are never the despotic master that the food addict slaves for. While the addict has a depraved, diseased, despotic, intollerably painful passion; the normal person experiences a healthy, mild, pleasant desire which is never painful and outrageous and which conforms perfectly to the real wants, the physiological needs, of the body. The difference is the same as that, between the "craving" of the inebriate for his alcohol and the desire of the normal man for a glass of pure water. *Normal demands are never painful.*

There are other reasons why a variety of foods should not be eaten besides the fact that they induce overeating. The greater the variety of food consumed at a meal, the more complicated and, consequently, less efficient, becomes the digestive process. Simple meals digest better and with less tax upon the digestive organs than complicated meals. Digestion is most efficient when but one food is eaten at a time. Where the limitations of the digestive enzymes are not respected, as is the case with millions, and no consideration is given to the proper combinations of foods, the more foods that are eaten at the meal the more complicated the digestive process becomes.

The reader will please bear in mind that we offer no objection to eating a variety of foods. We believe, on the contrary, in eating a wide variety of them. We are here discussing the evils of the common practice of trying to secure the whole variety at one meal. Properly managed, a variety of foods guarantees better nourishment than only a few foods.

Whole plants, or the total of the edible portions of particular plants, do not contain all the food factors required by man in correct correlations for his use. Only by eating a variety of plant foods, so selected that the total diet of fruits, nuts and green vegetables can supply all the food-factors required, can he be well and adequately nourished. The mono-diet is a fallacy, at least, so far as the higher animals and man are concerned. Variety we need, but not the whole variety at one meal.

To return to our main theme, that of overeating induced by great variety at meals, let us point out that it is practically impossible to avoid overeating so long as appetite is constantly tempted and *stimulated* by a great variety of foods. So long as we insist on having a great variety of foods at the meal, the evils of overeating will remain with us.

It is a good plan to serve one (at most two) cooked vegetables along with a salad and a protein or starch; or, better still serve the salad and protein or starch only and no cooked food. This kind of eating does not tempt to overeating.

Fruit is best eaten at a fruit meal and not too great a variety of fruits at a time. Three fruits at a meal should meet the demands of everyone.

Many people eat large quantities of bulky foods merely to "fill up." They are not "satisfied" unless they feel full. This is not necessary. It is not healthful. It does not improve function. *We ought to get away from the idea that our main object in life is to be forever filling up and emptying out again.*

Men who work hard or who work long hours insist that they require large quantities of food to meet their needs. They insist that they need foods that "stick to the ribs." They work hard and can't live on hay. Men who work hard do need more food than the idlers. Men who do physical work need more food than those who do mental work. But the differences in the food needs of these two classes are not as great as they suppose. The fact is, these men, who so loudly proclaim their need for so much food, are food drunkards. They habitually eat two, three and four times as much food as they actually use.

They reduce their energy by their overeating and poison themselves thereby at the same time. When they miss their accustomed food stimulus and feel weak, dizzy, or have pains, they mistake these morbid symptoms for an indication that they need the great quantities of *stimulating* foods they habitually eat. They are enervated and toxemic from overeating and mistake the symptoms of these for the normal demands of the body for nourishment.

These people suffer much, age early and die prematurely because of their overeating. Heart disease, arteriosclerosis, diabetes, Bright's disease, cancer, etc., finish them off years before they would reach the end if they ate prudently. These are the endings of those who live by "the belly's gospel of three squares plus and go by your appetite." These people should bear in mind Graham's words: *"A drunkard may reach old age, but a glutton, never."*

Enjoyment of Eating

CHAPTER XXVII

It is quite the custom to berate men and women for eating for "mere pleasure" instead of eating to supply the needs of the body. It is of course, true that the purpose of eating is to supply the body's nutritive needs, but eating should also be a pleasurable performance. All too often, however, we fail to extract due pleasure from our eating because we have forgotten how to eat. We do not taste any more—we merely swallow. Healthful eating requires that we shall taste to the fullest, each mouthful of food. To swallow our foods without proper mastication and in barbarious haste is to ruin our digestive organs and die of dyspepsia when we should be in the prime of life. It is also to miss the exquisite joys of eating.

The man of business who hurries to his dinner, hurries through it, and hurries back to his dimes, eats as a necessity and not as a pleasure. His dry goods, exchange bills and commercial speculations, his business avocations which puzzle his brain through the forenoon, are still in his head while he swallows his hasty meal. The sound of the cash register, as it receives the nickles and dimes, is sweet music to his ears; the delicious flavors and delightful aromas of nature's own foods are missed by him.

The school child or the physical worker who gets but half an hour for lunch, must hurry through his eating and to work or play, without time to masticate his food and certainly without an opportunity to enjoy his eating. Well do I recall one young man who could never take time to enjoy his food. He hurried through his meal, often snapping his fingers as he ate, so "nervous" was he about the loss of time from business. On one occasion he said to me: "I wish somebody would invent some concentrated foods that we could take as pills so that we would not have to waste time in eating." When eating is thought of as a waste of time and hurried through as this man rushed through his meals, it cannot be enjoyed.

We go to great lengths to cultivate our taste for music, art, beauty, etc., but neglect our taste for food. By this is not meant that we do not enjoy eating. It is all too often true that, we do too much eating because we like to eat. What is meant is that we do not cultivate that fine discriminating taste for foods that we do for music or art. Few people are able to discriminate and enjoy the fine flavors of foods—hence the almost universal use of such *irritants* as salt, pepper, sauces, spices, catsup, mustard, etc. We seem to enjoy quantity rather than quality, and irritation rather than fine, delicate flavors. Many people eat like the old hen, who swallows grain after grain of corn or kernel after kernel of wheat with no enjoyment of its taste, being satisfied with its bulk.

We should so cultivate our sense of taste that we can enjoy the flavors of foods as well as their bulk. To swallow food almost as soon as it is taken into the mouth is to deprive oneself of the enjoyment of its delicious flavors. To take time to thoroughly chew and insalivate foodstuffs, not only develops their flavors and affords opportunity to get ten to twenty times more enjoyment out of eating, but is assures better digestion. We can cultivate our sense of taste and learn to enjoy the fine delicate flavors of foods in the same way that we cultivate the sense of sight or that of hearing—*by exercise*. How do we learn to appreciate good music? By exercise of the tonal sense. We may learn to appreciate the finer flavors of our foods by exercise of the gustatory sense.

If a fruit, for example, is kept in the mouth until all of its delicious flavors, aromas and sweets have been yielded up and we have fully appreciated its richness, we soon acquire the ability to discriminate between the flavors of foods. In those who bolt their foods, who eat them piping hot or very cold, or who so disguise them with seasonings and condiments that their natural flavors are not discernable, the sense of taste is commonly so dormant that they are unable to tell the differences in flavor between one variety of apple and another variety of apple.

In the beautiful economy of nature the sense of taste is especially designed to relish most those particular foods that are in harmony with the constitutional nature of man. The normal, or unperverted sense of taste, will, therefore, derive the greatest enjoyment and the highest pleasure out of those foods to which man is constitutionally adapted, rather than out of the great mass of foodstuffs that are now eaten that do not fall within this range. Certain it is, that the normal taste will relish the natural flavors of foods much more than the *irritations* of condiments and spices.

The surest guarantee that one may fully enjoy one's food is a normal sense of taste and, fundamentally, this requires a normal condition of the physiological apparatus of taste. Anything and everything that blunts or perverts the sense of taste must inevitably detract from the normal and wholesome enjoyment of food.

Nerve endings in the tongue that are so benumbed by piping hot drinks and foods, or that are practically paralyzed from chronic nicotine poisoning and the heat of cigar, cigarette or pipe, or that are rendered temporarily useless by cold, lose their fine sensibilities and are powerless to discriminate between fine flavors and harsh ones. Indeed, they may be so palsied that they are unable to detect the finer flavors of foods. The callousing of the tongue, which guards against pain and irritation, prevents delicacy of nerve action, hence the gustatory apparatus of those who use hot tea and coffee, those who smoke, those who eat piping hot dishes, or who eat heavily condimented foods, those who habitually take cold drinks and iced foods, is in such an impaired condition that they can know very little of the deliciousness of foods. Especially are they likely to reject fruit because they do not relish it.

Pepper, mustard, vinegar, pungent spices, etc., and various drugs so *irritate* the taste buds, ultimately deadening them, both against the *irritant* and the finer flavors of foods, that, all power of discrimination is lost. To such a sense of taste all uncondimented foods are flat, dull, insipid. The owner of such an impaired gustatory sense does not enjoy natural foods in their unseasoned state. The fine delicate flavors with which nature has savored her foods are missed by him. As he continues the use of his condiments, his tobacco, his drugs, etc., he is forced to use more and more or stronger and stronger condiments in order that he may "relish" his food at all.

Many years ago, I observed that tobacco users do not like fruit. The successful use of fruit diets of various kinds in remedying various drug habits, indicates that the use of fruit and the use of drugs is incompatible. It is extremely difficult to continue to use both varieties of substances. I have repeatedly called attention to these facts, both in my writings and my lectures. It is interesting to record that I have recently found reference to this same fact in *Hygienic* literature published in 1849. Tobacco using incapacities the users for the enjoyment of the deliciousness of fruits; they deriving their greatest satisfaction from the quantity of the food eaten rather than from its fine flavors. They commonly require that their foods be rendered "hot' by spices or something that "burns" such as mustard, pepper, etc. As these things are comparatively devoid of flavor, but little gustatory enjoyment is derived from eating seasoned foods.

Hygienists declared in 1849 that "probably more than anything else, tobacco is ruinous to the nerves of taste. This powerfully biting *stimulant* in the mouth for hours and days together—a fresh quid taken as soon as the old one is disgorged—the mouth kept in one burning fever of excitement—all its nerves saturated with tobacco juice, so that they are obliged to harden themselves against this foreign enemy—they become blunted to anything like richness of flavor. They may tell the difference between sweet and sour, but cannot enjoy either, and are comparatively dead." Tobacco users, even those who smoke (the foregoing quotation refers particularly to the practice of chewing tobacco), thus debar themselves from almost all of the pleasures of eating, especially do they deprive themselves of the pleasures derived from the many varieties of delicious flavors in natural foods. The tobacco user does not know what rich goodness there is in foods and he (or she) can never know until the poison-vice is discontinued and sufficient time has elapsed for the tongue to slough off its callous and for its palsied nerves to be revived.

Drs. Ada R. Hall and A. F. Blakeslee had smokers taste a chemical known as PTC, before and after smoking. After smoking 75% required a much stronger solution before they could taste it at all, and 20% a weaker solution. The main point was that 58% required an hour before the taste sense returned to its pre-smoking status, so they could taste the same strength of PTC as before smoking. This is thought to be probably true of foods, also.

Apparently no tests were made with foods, so that I cannot contend that my observations have been verified *scientifically*—that is, by the much vaunted "scientific method." The tests that were made are not of a character to determine accurately the truth of my observations. They show merely that the use of tobacco lessens the acuteness of the sense of taste in most smokers and "heightens" it in a few. This effect was apparently temporary, lasting an hour in the majority of individuals tested. My own observations have been on the lasting results of habitual smoking and not on the temporary results following one smoke.

In saying that tobacco users do not like fruits, I imply much more than a mere temporary lessening of the acuteness of the sense of taste and smell—much of what we think of as taste of food is really smell of the food. I do not mean merely, that they do not taste the food, but that they do not relish the taste of it. Now, lest some tobacco user write me and say that I am wrong because he likes cranberry sauce, or another write me and say that I am wrong because he likes blue berries, or something of this nature, let me say that the degree of loss of relish for fruits varies with individual tobacco users and varies with particular fruits.

The tests made by Hall and Blakeslee, show, not so much a change as a weakening of the sense of taste. My observations indicate an actual change of taste. The tobacco user relishes other foods. Perhaps his relish, even for these, is not very keen, due to the weakening of the sense of taste.

Tobacco is not the only drug used habitually by Americans that weakens and changes their sense of taste. Salt and various hot condiments and "relishes," and alcohol do the same thing. After these things have been used for some time the power to sense the fine delicate flavors in natural foods is completely lost, so that such foods are dull, flat, insipid to the user of these substances. He is unable to understand how anybody can eat foods without the "seasoning." He does not realize that the trouble is not with the foods, but with himself. He has so numbed, blunted and paralyzed his taste buds that they are no longer able to detect the fine delicate flavors and have lost their powers of discrimination. Some of them I have known have lost their power to detect bitter substances, even the bitterness of quinine not registering. These substances stand in the way of real enjoyment of his foods.

One fallacy contained in the conclusions reached from these tests, is that the sense of taste "returned to normal" after the lapse of an hour or less, in those tested. This implies that the taste of the smoker is normal, except while he is smoking and for a brief period thereafter. This assumption is far from true. The smoker's senses of taste and smell are, alike, much impaired. They are not normal. The taste of the smoker is not as acute as that of the non-smoker.

It is not as discriminating in its detection of various flavors. It is not able to appreciate the finer and more delicate flavors in foods. In the case of fruits, fruit flavors that are relished by non-smokers are likely to be positively distasteful to the smoker.

While these tests were made on smokers, I have observed that the use of tobacco in the form of chewing tobacco and snuff has the same effect upon the sense of taste, perhaps not as much upon the sense of smell, as smoking. Indeed, I think it is demonstrable that chewing tobacco impairs the sense of taste even more than does smoking.

To assume that smokers have a normal sense of taste which returns to normal in a brief period after they throw away their butts, is to assume that which is definitely not so. It is right, perhaps, to say that the chronic impairment of their sense of taste is aggravated temporarily by each smoke, and that the temporary aggravation is "recovered" from shortly after the smoking has ceased. To recover from the chronic impairment that has resulted from habitual smoking, it is necessary to cease smoking and refrain from the practice for an extended period—weeks and months.

I saw no mention of "controls" in these experiments. Where were the "controls"? Were no tests made on non-smokers? How are the effects of smoking upon the sense of taste to be fully explored if no tests are made on non-smokers? A careful comparison of the sense of taste of both groups is essential to full understanding of the matter. If this is done, the experimenters will find that smoking changes and does not merely weaken the taste for foods. They will discover, also, that the smoker does not have a normal sense of taste to return to an hour after he has had his smoke. I suggest, also that they test the changes in the sense of taste in a man as this slowly returns to normal after he abandons smoking. Finally, I would suggest that foods, and not chemicals, be used in the tests. This latter suggestion may not be "scientific." It may be very unscientific to test the taste for foods by using foods.

Recent tests made by psychologist Katheryn Langwill revealed that women could distinguish finer differences than could men in four basic tastes: sweet, salt, sour and bitter. Her tests showed that one-half of both men and women preferred "moderately sweet and salty" foods. More women than men preferred extremely salty and sour foods. Over one-half of the men liked slightly sour foods. These tests and their results are without meaning if the matter of perversion and taste impairment caused by alcohol, tobacco, condiments, heat, cold, etc., are not given due consideration. To be conclusive, such tests would have to be made on men and women with normal sense of taste, not on those who have impaired their sense of taste by years of abuse. It should be obvious that that individual and that sex whose taste apparatus has been most abused will have the least power of discrimination; that is, will be least able to detect finer differences. It is probable that there is no difference in the taste perceptions of normal individuals of either sex. The different habits of the two sexes must account for much of the differences in capacities seen in them.

The sense of taste may be so nearly completely paralyzed that only the strongest and most pungent substances can be tasted. Mild, delicate flavors are not tasted at all. In those individuals whose sense of taste is thus impaired, no pleasure would be derived from eating unspiced foods. They would have a "preference" for very hot, or very sour, or very sweet substances. How foolish to test men and women with varying degrees of palsied taste in an effort to determine which of the sexes can taste flavors better! This, however, is just what we should expect of a psychologist, for psychologists have the bad habit of accepting things-as-they-unfortunately-are as the normal state of things. They never think that there may be anything wrong with our present mode of life and the conditions under which it is lived.

The pernicious idea that the cultivation and gratification of morbid appetancies constitutes the cultivation of taste is productive of much harm. Equally harmful is the idea that the cultivation of taste consists essentially in the multiplication of human wants without reference to the purposes accomplished through the instrumentality of such wants. Weakness and perversion with the resulting suffering inevitably flow from such false cultivation. It is analogous to cultivating a patch of noxious weeds instead of a beautiful garden of flowers.

In proportion to the intensity of every passion is the capacity for refinement and for degradation. The hardest steel bears the sharpest edge. The densest metals are the most ductile and malleable. The sense of taste may be cultivated and refined, or it may be abused, neglected and degraded. The choice is ours.

How to Eat

CHAPTER XXVIII,

Gastronomy is the art of dining well when the table is set to one's liking. *Gastrosophy* is far more than this. It is the harmonious interlocking of production, preparation and consumption of food. Gastrosophy is the grand field where the labors and arts of the garden and kitchen, the orchards, vineyards and conservatories all meet and mingle and where the luxury of appreciation has been earned by the labors which have preceded it.

The discrimination of specific adaptations of different foodstuffs to certain organisms and constitutions, belongs also to that sphere of science which we term *gastrosophy*. The first step in the establishment of a valid gastrosophy is the determination of the normal or constitutional dietetic character of man.

Hunger is the organic or assimilative *passion* in which the wants of the body are reflected in the form of distinct mouth and throat sensation, often by means of a distinct desire for a particular food. True hunger is rarely indiscriminate. It is not a blind impulse to eat, but a definite desire to eat certain foods. Real hunger is earned by the labors which have preceded it and is not prompted by the clock. *Appetite*, which is a counterfit hunger, is commonly finicky, indiscriminate, unearned and periodic. It relates to habit rather than to need.

The first rule of eating should be: *Wait upon hunger*. One should eat when hungry and only when hungry. Then, he should eat sufficient to satisfy the demands of hunger. Nothing is to be gained by eating beyond the normal demands of the body for food. Eating should be an exquisite pleasure, but pleasure should not be the end and aim of eating.

If you follow the practice of eating when hungry and only when hungry, there will be no regular meal times and there will be no eating between meals. If your work is such that you must set aside certain periods of the day for eating and eat at these times, without reference to hunger, then, you should by all means abstain from eating between meals. Likewise, you should not eat in the evening before retiring. This does not mean that it is not well to go to bed "on a full stomach." It simply means that if you have had your regular meals, there is no need for an added meal after the theater or after the card game or the social chat. Eating as a social function, should also be avoided. All of these types of eating not only lead to over eating, but they interfere with the digestion of the regular meals.

The second rule of correct eating should be: *Eat all the food required to satisfy hunger and then cease*. Overeating carries its own penalties. In civilized life we make a merit of gorging everything set before us and it is even considered a grave misdemeanor in children to be "choicey" about their food. Mothers and fathers, physicians and nurses are supposed to know what best to prepare for them. What business have they with instincts! Why should they have preferences; how dare they attempt to choose? Does not the adult know what is proper for them and when they should eat? Does he not even know how much they should eat? True, it may be, that, the adult does not know how to feed himself, but he certainly knows all there is to know about the feeding of children!

Although for thousands of years over-nutrition and its results have puzzled the authorities, it is known definitely that wholesome food taken in too great quantities becomes a dissipation, both enervating and poisoning the eater. In conditions of surfeit the parts of the organism lack the "stimulus" for work, both physiological and biological. Surfeit and rich fare "stimulate" in pathological directions. For example, there seems to be a hereditary transmission of an arthritic tendency (diathesis) which arises out of habitual surfeit.

The body is duly nourished only when the proper food which has been eaten is also properly digested. If the functions of digestion are impaired so that the food eaten is inadequately digested, then, no food, however nutritious and well fitted to meet the needs of the organism, will afford healthy sustenance to the body. When from overeating, for example, digestion becomes impaired so that food ceases to be nutritious, the more the individual eats, the more he is poisoned, rather than nourished, by his food. Want of nourishment results from lack of power to digest as often as from lack of food.

Properly speaking a meal consists of two elements, a spiritual and a material food. Since a cheerful tone of mind .and joyous associations enable us not only to enjoy our foods more but to digest them better, friendship, mirth, wit, good stories, love and absence of distractions, irritations, bitterness, etc., compose the spiritual essence of a good meal. If the eater is not fully at ease, if there are family quarrels at the dining table, if there is officiousness of the head of the family as to the eating of the other members, if gloom and depression hang like a dark pall over the table, the food will not be enjoyed nor will it be efficiently digested.

Perhaps the best time and place to tell funny stories is at the dining table at meal time. It is far better for everyone around the table to tell a funny joke or story at the table and get everyone to laughing, than to come to the table grouchy and make every one tense and "nervous." Laughter promotes relaxation and ease. At the table let peace and joy reign supreme. This should be the rule of life.

Fatigue, pain, fear, grief, anxiety, depression, tension, anger, self-pity, inflammation and fever and similar emotional and physical states cause the fountains of digestive juices to dry up and the normal movements of the digestive tract to slow down or to be altogether suspended. When one eats in any one of these states one invites indigestion and its consequent discomfort and poisoning. Our rules should be:

If not comfortable from one meal to the next miss the meal.

If there is pain, fever, inflammation, miss the meal—miss as many meals as required for these to pass.

If under emotional strain—if angry, grieved, depressed, worried, anxious, etc.—miss one or more meals until emotional poise has been regained.

If fatigued, rest a bit before eating. There is nothing like a period of rest and relaxation to restore functional vigor to the tired man.

Man is equipped with a chewing apparatus. Chewing food breaks it up into fine particles so that the digestive juices may get to it. Chewing insures thorough insalivation of food. It also assures that the food shall be tasted and this is important in the adaptation of the digestive juices to the character of the food. Chewing and tasting food enable us to really enjoy our food. Swallowing food without tasting it means that we do not derive due pleasure from eating. If food is well chewed and not bolted, we enjoy it more and digest it better, so that we are better nourished. Thorough chewing of food will also enable us to tell when we have had enough. Our rule should be: *Chew your food, your stomach has no teeth.*

The popular American habit of chewing gum definitely retards the digestion of food, particularly in the stomach and is no "aid to digestion," as it is frequently advertised to be. Gum chewing depresses gastric acidity for an hour or more. Gum chewing after meals, and particularly after protein meals, is definitely detrimental to all who indulge in the practice.

Water, according to the principles of *Natural Hygiene,* is the only true drink. All other liquids that are taken as drinks are either foods (milk, fruit juices, etc.) or poisons (coffee, tea, cocoa, alcoholic liquors, etc.) and should be taken as foods or abstained from as poisons. So-called "soft drinks" are not true drinks and are not *soft.* Made of artificially colored water (colored with coal-tar dyes) to which synthetic flavors and phosphoric acid have been added, sweetened with white sugar and then given a dose of some popular poison, such as caffeine, they are definitely harmful substances and the wise person will abstain from them at all times and under all circumstances.

Thirst is the indication that water is required. This has reference to genuine thirst and not to a fictitious thirst that is caused by salt, condiments, etc. Our rule should be: *drink when thirsty and only when thirsty.* But, we should not drink with meals, nor soon thereafter. Water dilutes the digestive juices, passes from the stomach in a very few minutes and takes the juices along with it, so that the food is left without adequate juice to carry on the work of digestion. Digestion goes on in the stomach for variable periods of time after meals and the meal should not be inundated with water at any stage of the digestive process.

All the water desired should be taken ten to twenty minutes before meals.

All the water desired may be taken thirty minutes after a fruit meal.

All the water desired may be taken two hours after a starch meal.

All the water desired may be taken four hours after a protein meal.

The rule not to drink with meals should be understood to apply to all such liquids as coffee, tea, fruit and vegetable juices, etc., that are commonly taken with meals. If it is desirable to have fruit or vegetable juices added to the diet, these should be taken fifteen to twenty minutes before the meal, or at some interval sufficiently distant from the meal that it offers no interference with the digestion of the meal.

But little space may be devoted to food combining in this book. Readers desiring to learn the facts and principles underlying the following rules for food combining, should study my *Food Combining Made Easy.* The rules are:

1.—Eat acids and starches at separate meals.

2.—Eat protein foods and carbohydrate foods at separate meals.

3.—Eat but one concentrated protein food at a meal.

4.—Eat proteins and acids at separate meals.

5.—Eat fats and proteins at separate meals.

6.—Eat sugars and proteins at separate meals.

7.—Eat melons alone.

8.—Take milk alone or let it alone. (For the vegetarian who takes no milk, this rule is to be observed in feeding milk to infants and small children).

Desserts are tid-bits, or confections, that are eaten after one has eaten more than enough. They combine with nothing and are best omitted from the bill-of-fare.

Planning Meals

"Choose what is best; habit will soon render it agreeable and easy," advised Pythagoras. We may easily learn to relish any wholesome food, even, although it does not appeal to our gustatory sense when first taken. It is very unfortunate that most people will not make the little effort required to acquire a liking for foods that, when first tried, do not appeal to their senses of taste and smell. A man that will take much time, make repeated efforts and suffer much in acquiring a "liking" for tobacco, or for beer, will forever refuse to eat celery because the first time he tried it, he did not like it. A woman tries her first avocado and exclaims: "It tastes like a mouthful of lard." Thereafter she never tries avocados any more. Another person tries his first mango and does not like its taste. Forever after he refuses mangos. But he can drink coffee by the cups full. If such people will follow the advice of Pythagoras they will soon find that they can learn to relish and enjoy any and all wholesome foods.

It is unfortunate that habit also renders "agreeable and easy" that which is not best. We take some red pepper into our mouth and stomach with food. It occasions a strong, almost unbearable "burning" in the mouth, throat, stomach, intestine and in the rectum, as it is expelled. Due to the irritation thus occasioned, peristalsis is increased and the meal is sent along the digestive tract without being digested and is expelled in much less than normal time. To allay the "burning," we take much water into the mouth and stomach. The whole experience is very disagreable and there is every indication that the body rebels against a non-usable and injurious substance. But we persist in using it until we get to the point where we can use it in liberal quantities with but an "agreeable" stimulation (irritation) and no rush takes place in sending the meal through the digestive tract. Now we discover that our foods do not taste well without the pepper. Yet it is nonetheless useless and injurious and is still rejected by the body. Thickening and hardening (callous) of the lining membranes of the digestive tract have blunted the irritating effects of the pepper and rendered less sensitive the nerve endings in these membranes. Digestion is also crippled and the whole organism has been enervated by the use of the pepper (the same is true of all other condiments), but, because there has been, as a result of the use of the piquant condiment, a blunting of the sense of taste, we now find ourselves unable to detect the fine, delicate flavors in our foods and can relish them only if they are filled with pepper. We continue to eat pepper and to gradually increase the amount used, as our taste function continues to deteriorate. Life without pepper is now unthinkable. What a predicament we have gotten ourselves into!

If you have cultivated such unwholesome eating habits, these should be abandoned at once and permanently. Do not try to "taper off," for you will fail. Give up the condiments at once and in full and be assured that, although you do not enjoy your food at first, nature will soon slough off the callous and restore your normal sensitivity, so that, you may again appreciate the delicious flavors with which she has savored her foods. Soon you will discover fine delicate flavors in your foods that you have forgotten are there.

When, in the hardness and rebellion of your old perversions, you turn back to your old habits, and it is always easy to return to them, to your condiments, flesh-pots and poison-vices, practices which were acquired in the days of ignorance and incoherence, you must know that you injure yourself and weaken the very foundations of life. When you have determined to abandon the old habits, let nothing deter you from carrying out this determination. The effort to break the old habits and to establish new ones will be a short one and success will be well rewarded. Adopt no compromise plan, but become a true radical in this matter and completely uproot the old harmful practices. You'll fail if you convince yourself that you lack will power (you have as much will power as anyone else), for the struggle will not be an easy one. You can succeed, if you will but make a real effort.

The menus presented in this chapter contain no compromises. They are intended for those who desire to eat only biologically legitimate foods and to eat them in proper combinations. No limits have been placed on quantities, for the reason that some people require more than others in order to be well nourished. Each reader of this book will determine how much of any food he will eat. If he finds himself losing weight on the menus presented, he will not add other foods to the menus, thus complicating the digestive process, but will simply eat more of the same foods.

In the Nov. 1950 issue of *Nature's Path* W. R. Raymond discusses the relative values of animal and seed proteins. He makes several references to "meat substitutes" during the course of the article. He states that "the soybean has been highly recommended as a meat substitute. However, after long research, the writer has found that sesame seed proteins are far superior to soybean protein as a meat substitute, for they are not only more easily digested, but, when properly prepared, they provide a vegetable meat which looks, tastes and smells more like real meat than soybean meat substitutes do." He thus gives expression to the viewpoint of the great majority of vegetarians.

The true vegetarian does not look for and does not want, for he knows that he does not need a "meat substitute." He knows that in giving up the flesh foods he gives up the substitute. Why shall vegetarians continue to prepare concoctions of various kinds that look, taste and smell like flesh? I submit that they do this because, emotionally, at least, they have never weaned themselves from their flesh diet. If flesh forms no part of man's normal diet, then a substitute for flesh is not needed. If it does form a normal part of man's diet, then the vegetarian is running counter to his own nature and contrary to his own best interests, when he refrains from eating flesh.

Raymond gives instructions for making "milk," "cream" and dressing of nuts and seeds, the products "resembling corresponding dairy products quite closely." This is another of those all too common efforts to make the vegetarian diet resemble the carnivorous diet. Honesty and consistency will cause us either to abandon dairy products and not try to imitate them, or to use dairy products. The true vegetarian will not seek to imitate the animal food diet.

Many of the meat substitutes sold in the market are indigestible combinations of cereals and legumes. They are cooked, canned, stored and thus greatly deteriorated. Many of the concoctions that are made at home—mock turkey, mock chicken, etc.—are also indigestible combinations. Why not simplify your diet? This will assure you better nutrition and will relieve the wife of a great burden of unnecessary work in preparing meals. Take her out of the kitchen and let her devote more time to other activities.

One of the most important parts of any diet is the salad. A large salad of uncooked vegetables should be taken with each protein and each starch meal. The "salads" served in hotels and restaurants and made in the average home are travesties on the name. Egg salad, potato salad, shrimp salad, and the like do not merit the name salad. The addition of pickles and dressings to these abominable mixtures only serves to make them less desirable. Commonly bad combinations in themselves, they do not combine with the balance of the meal. Dressings made of oil and vinegar or oil and lemon juice, or of oil alone or of lemon juice alone, or dressings of cream or of nut creams, etc., not only smother the flavors of the salad, but combine poorly with the balance of the meal. Salads are best eaten plain, this is to say, without dressing of any kind.

Have a large salad. This is important, for in the fresh, uncooked ingredients of the salad is an abundance of minerals, vitamins and enzymes that are essential to adequate nutrition of young and old alike. Do not shred, chop and cut up the ingredients of the salad. The following salads are but samples intended to guide you in making your own salads:

Half a head of lettuce, celery and cucumber. (Do not peel the cucumber).

Half a head of lettuce, celery and cabbage.
Half a head of lettuce, celery and tomato (whole).
Half a head of lettuce, cabbage and bell pepper (green or ripe).
Half a head of lettuce, French endive and tomato (whole).
Half a head of lettuce, spinach and fresh tender okra.
Cabbage, cucumber and radishes.

If it is desired, a sprig or two of parsley may be added to any or all of these salads. They may be arranged artistically, and by the addition of a little color, such as a little red sweet pepper, may be made to appeal to the eyes as well as to the sense of taste. No salt should be added to them, as they are abundant in organic salts. Keep them simple and do not throw a dozen or more vegetables together haphazardly in making a salad.

The following menus are also intended as guides to you in preparing your own menus. They are properly combined and if you will study them carefully, in connection with the rules for food combining that were given in the preceding chapter, you will be able to prepare your own properly combined meals, or to select properly combined foods wherever you may be. Meals, like salads, should be simple. Seven course and twenty-one course dinners, in which everything "from soup to nuts" is served, are indigestible combinations that cause trouble.

No desserts are included in these meals. Desserts are luxuries—tidbits—and the more they are indulged, the more they undermine health. Dessert eating is always that much too much, besides always being wrong combinations with all the other foods of the meal. Often indigestible themselves, desserts render difficult the digestion of any meal. Dr. Tilden's advice about eating pie may well be applied to other forms of dessert. He said that if you must have pie, have it alone and miss the next meal. Gladstone's secret of long life— "plain eating and high thinking"—deserves a worthy place on the wall of every dining room. Eat right, drink only water, be merry and tomorow we live again.

I have prepared the first two weeks menus to cover foods that are in season in Spring and Summer and the second two week's menus to cover foods in season during the Fall and Winter season.

MENUS FOR SPRING AND SUMMER

MONDAY

BREAKFAST	LUNCH	DINNER
Cherries	Vegetable Salad	Vegetable Salad
Plums	Cooked Spinach	Chard
Apricots	Fresh Corn	Okra
	Carrots	Nuts

TUESDAY

BREAKFAST	LUNCH	DINNER
Canteloupe	Vegetable Salad	Vegetable Salad
	Green Beans	Spinach
	Beet Tops	Okra
	Baked Potatoes	Avocado

WEDNESDAY

BREAKFAST	LUNCH	DINNER
Grapefruit	Vegetable Salad	Vegetable Salad
	Turnip Greens	Green Squash
	Steamed Turnips	Fresh Corn
	Baked Beans	Sunflower Seed

—176—

THURSDAY

BREAKFAST	LUNCH	DINNER
Watermelon	Vegetable Salad	Vegetable Salad
	Broccoli	Kale
	Asparagus	Squash
	Sweet Potatoes	Pignolias

FRIDAY

BREAKFAST	LUNCH	DINNER
Nectarines	Vegetable Salad	Vegetable Salad
Bananas	Spinach	Beet Tops
Cherries	Carrots	Okra
	Cauliflower	Mixed Nuts

SATURDAY

BREAKFAST	LUNCH	DINNER
Honey Dew	Peaches	Vegetable Salad
	Plums	Chard
	Apricots	Green Beans
		Avocado

SUNDAY

BREAKFAST	LUNCH	DINNER
Watermelon	Vegetable Salad	Cherries
	Yellow Squash	Nectarines
	Spinach	Bananas
	Sunflower Seed	

MONDAY

BREAKFAST	LUNCH	DINNER
Oranges	Vegetable Salad	Vegetable Salad
	Kohlrabi	Okra
	Turnip Tops	Yellow Wax Beans
	Carrots	Peanuts

TUESDAY

BREAKFAST	LUNCH	DINNER
Peaches	Vegetable Salad	Vegetable Salad
Plums	Okra	Asparagus
Fresh Figs	Kale	Eggplant (baked)
	Baked Potatoes	Brazil Nuts

WEDNESDAY

BREAKFAST	LUNCH	DINNER
Watermelon	Apricots	Vegetable Salad
	Cherries	Chard
	Bananas	Green Beans
		Pecans

THURSDAY

BREAKFAST	LUNCH	DINNER
Mangos	Vegetable Salad	Vegetable Salad
Peaches	Turnip Greens	Beet Greens
Plums	Carrots	Steamed Turnips
	Coconut	Avocado

FRIDAY

BREAKFAST	LUNCH	DINNER
Canteloupe	Bananas	Vegetable Salad
	Cherries	Kale
	Nectarines	Asparagus
		Pistachio Nuts

SATURDAY

BREAKFAST	LUNCH	DINNER
Peaches	Vegetable Salad	Vegetable Salad
Plums	Okra	Green Beans
Bananas	Spinach	Yellow Squash
	Baked Beans	Mixed Nuts

SUNDAY

BREAKFAST	LUNCH	DINNER
Watermelon	Vegetable Salad	Mango
	Asparagus	Cherries
	Kale	Apricots
	Cashew Nuts	

MENUS FOR THE FALL AND WINTER

MONDAY

BREAKFAST	LUNCH	DINNER
Pear	Vegetable Salad	Vegetable Salad
Apple	Chinese Cabbage	Spinach
Grapes	String Beans	Steamed Beets
	Baked Hubbard Squash	Sunflower Seed

TUESDAY

BREAKFAST	LUNCH	DINNER
Grapes	Vegetable Salad	Vegetable Salad
Apple	Kale	Green Beans
Dried Figs	Green Squash	Spinach
	Caladium Roots	Avocado

WEDNESDAY

BREAKFAST	LUNCH	DINNER
Persimmons	Vegetable Salad	Vegetable Salad
Grapes	Broccoli	Beet Greens
Dates	Beet Greens	Baked Eggplant
	Baked Squash	Pecans

THURSDAY

BREAKFAST	LUNCH	DINNER
Oranges	Vegetable Salad	Vegetable Salad
Grapefruit	Kale	Chard
	String Beans	Asparagus
	Yams	Peanuts

FRIDAY

BREAKFAST	LUNCH	DINNER
Persimmons	Vegetable Salad	Vegetable Salad
Grapes	Broccoli	Baked Eggplant
Apple	Spinach	Green Beans
	Baked Potatoes	Mixed Nuts

SATURDAY

BREAKFAST	LUNCH	DINNER
Grapefruit	Persimmons	Vegetable Salad
	Pear	Kale
	Dates	Yellow Squash
		Avocado

SUNDAY

BREAKFAST	LUNCH	DINNER
Oranges	Vegetable Salad	Persimmon
Grapefruit	Asparagus	Apple
	Chard	Grapes
	Mixed Nuts	

MONDAY

BREAKFAST	LUNCH	DINNER
Grapes	Vegetable Salad	Vegetable Salad
Pear	Spinach	Green Squash
Dates	Baked Cauliflower	Beet Greens
		Sunflower Seed

TUESDAY

BREAKFAST	LUNCH	DINNER
Persimmons	Vegetable Salad	Vegetable Salad
Grapes	Kale	Spinach
Apple	Green Beans	Asparagus
	Yams	Baked Beans

WEDNESDAY

BREAKFAST	LUNCH	DINNER
Grapefruit	Vegetable Salad	Vegetable Salad
	Carrots	Baked Eggplant
	Green Peas	Yellow Wax Beans
	Baked Potatoes	Pecans

THURSDAY

BREAKFAST	LUNCH	DINNER
Honey Dew Melon	Vegetable Salad	Vegetable Salad
	Beet Tops	Chard
	Asparagus	Yellow Squash
	Jerusalem Artichokes	Brazil Nuts

FRIDAY

BREAKFAST	LUNCH	DINNER
Persimmons	Vegetable Salad	Vegetable Salad
Grapes	Green Beans	Kale
Dates	Turnip Greens	Green Squash
	Wholegrain Bread	Mixed Nuts

SATURDAY

BREAKFAST	LUNCH	DINNER
Grapes	Vegetable Salad	Vegetable Salad
Apple	Green Peas	Spinach
Pear	Broccoli	Asparagus
	Caladium Root	Avocado

SUNDAY

BREAKFAST	LUNCH	DINNER
Grapefruit	Vegetable Salad	Persimmons
Oranges	Beet Tops	Grapes
	Green Beans	Apple
	Pine Nuts	Dates

Preparing For Winter

CHAPTER XXX

"In time of peace prepare for war," runs an old adage. In Spring, Summer and Fall, when days are warm and skies are clear, prepare for winter, when the days will be cold and the skies cloudy. This is the way of life, and those who give themselves a chance may face next winter without fear and dread.

The student of nature will recognize at once, that the lower animals that do not migrate, but that remain at home to face the winter months, prepare for the coming period of inclemency by laying up, either within their own bodies or without, stores of appropriate food supplies. Unlike man, they do not deliberately dissipate these supplies, once winter has set in.

Those of my readers who are not acquainted with the *Laws of Life* as explained in chapter 6 of Vol. 1 of the *Hygienic System,* are, perhaps, ignorant of the *Law of Special Economy* there formulated thus: *The Vital organism, under favorable conditions, stores up all excess of vital funds, above the current expenditure, as a reserve fund to be employed in a time of special need.*

Organisms capitalize the results of the joint work of their several organs and physiological systems in the form of capacities and valuable stored substances. They may learn to use this stored capital, which they have woven into their fabric and built into their flesh and bone and blood, in the interest of the whole organism, or in doing useful work; or they may consume it in wasteful expenditure of one kind or another; or they may use it under circumstances that place the body under special or unusual stress.

Stored capacities and substances constitute the reserve power of an organism; power held out of activity under ordinary conditions to be used under extraordinary conditions—acute crises, poisoning, prolonged or intense cold, prolonged or intense heat, extreme or prolonged exertion, profound emotional experiences, shock, or other emergency and stress.

In the North, winters are long, cold and more or less sunless. Before winter ends there is much suffering attributable in part to lack of sunlight. Long winters exhaust the meager reserves carried by most civilized beings. If reserves were greater, exhaustion would not occur and trouble would not develop.

The body does not store up sunshine. It stores up substances produced by the aid of sunshine. Not vitamin D alone, but other materials are synthesized in the body with the aid of the sun's rays and the surpluses of these are stored in the tissues as reserve capital for times of stringency. If these sun-kissed reserves are abundant and not wasted they will carry the individual through a long, sunless winter.

Before they can carry the man, woman, or child through the winter, they must exist. They must have been stored up during the seasons of sun and warmth. The individual must have made full and proper use of the sun while it was available. The man who has spent the sunny months indoors, or who has clad himself in such manner that the sun has been excluded from contact with his body, will posses no such reserve with which to meet the demands of life in winter.

That person who has had plenty of sun, but who has dissipated his reserves, will also lack the needed stored substances with which to meet the winter. Reserves are dissipated by alcohol, tea, coffee, tobacco and all other forms of poisoning. Toxemia dissipates reserves. The organism that must ceaselessly use it substances in neutralizing, detoxicating and resisting poisons will not be able to store up ample reserves. Reserves are dissipated by all forms of excess and dissipation and by overworked emotions. They are wasted by a denatured diet; which, while failing to supply sufficient amounts of some elements of nutrition, force the body to employ part of its own stored capital to compensate for the deficiencies in the diet. Late hours, over work, loss of sleep, sexual excess—these all consume the body's reserves and deplete its physiological capital.

The best preparation with which to meet long, cold, cloudy winters, is a sensible, natural mode of living during the warm, sunny months and sensible living during the winter. Reserves that have been stored by the organism during a summer of prudent living may be quickly dissipated by excesses, indulgences, dissipations and wrong foods in the winter.

There would be no great increase in pneumonia and "other respiratory diseases" in February, in northern latitudes, if intelligence were used in our summer and winter living. If during the warm months we live in a manner that enables the body to store up an abundance of reserve substances and, if in the winter, we live in a manner to conserve these reserves and stretch them out as far as possible, winter ills will be less common and of little account. Indeed, there need be no winter ills.

In winter, especially in the small towns and cities, there is likely to be a derth of fresh fruits and vegetables. People in general tend to fall back on a diet lacking in many essential requirements and thus consume their meager stored reserves at a much faster rate than these would be consumed on a better diet.

Even in the small towns, apples, oranges, cabbage and a few other fresh vegetables and fruits are to be had in winter and, if used, these will help to greatly stretch out the stored reserves. In the larger cities, fruits and vegetables are usually plentiful in winter and, though often higher in price than at other seasons, are cheaper than doctor's bills, drug bills, nurse's bills, surgeon's bill, and loss of time from work due to illness—cheaper by far than undertaker's bills.

If the money regularly spent on tobacco, tea, coffee, chocolate, alcohol, soda-fountain slops and other popular poisons were spent, instead, on fruits and vegetables, a dual saving of reserves would result. Not alone would there be less deficiency in the diet to be compensated for by the reserves, but the reserves regularly employed in resisting, neutralizing and detoxicating these poisons would be saved.

Conservation of the body's energies and stored substances is the secret of reserve strength with which to meet, resist and successfully endure or overcome the emergencies of life, whatever these emergencies may be. Dissipating the body's energies and stored substances is the sure way to weakness, lost resistance, illness and death. Men and women who waste their substance in riotous living and in the conventionally approved forms of dissipation must keep ever in mind that "if we dance we must pay the fiddler."

The normal body draws upon its reserves so easily and readily that we seem not to be injured by our deficiencies and excesses. The body continues to meet our over drafts on the bank of vitality by invading its reserve funds so that we seem to be "doing all right." We are fooled by our apparent impunity. "We never miss the water 'till the well runs dry."

Intelligent and informed men and women will not be fooled by an apparent protracted impunity. They will know that repeated raids upon their reserves will exhaust them, even if, on the surface, they appear to be inexhaustible. Conservation of the forces of life is the great secret of power in reserve. Cease wasting your energies and substances.

During these days of day-light-saving, millions of people get away from their work early enough in the afternoon to get a sunbath each day before sundown. At the beach, on the roof of your apartment house, in the garden, even on the front lawn (in a bathing suit), in your room before an open window, or anywhere that you can get the sun without offending the super-sensitive eyes of prudish old Dame Grundy, will do for your sunbath. Put the children out on the beach, the green lawn or on the apartment roof. Be ready for winter when it comes around again.

Hygienic Care of The Sick

CHAPTER XXXI

Natural Hygiene, as distinguised from the spurious hygiene fostered by the schools of so-called healing, is a system of mind-body care, both in health and in sickness, based on a practical recognition and systematic carrying out of the organic laws of life in their entireness, as these are developed and explained by physiological and biological science. It is the employment, according to well-defined laws and demonstrable principles of nature, of materials, conditions and influences that have normal relations to life, in the preservation and restoration of health.

Natural Hygienists maintain that the aid given the sick, to be real and lasting rather than illusory and transient, must be founded upon the primary laws of life, as unfolded by physiology and biology, and reliance must be imposed upon a systematic application of the identical means, modified according to circumstances and need, that are requisite for maintaining the body in a state of vigorous health. *Hygienic* care of the well and the sick is reliance upon the normal elements of healthy life.

The *Natural Hygienist* seeks to restore health in the sick by the identical means that preserve health in the well, rather than by means that are well known to produce disease in the well. Integral to *Natural Hygiene* and forming the very basis upon which its remedial care is founded, is the principle that only those substances and means that are constitutionally adapted to the use of the human organism can be of use to it in a state of illness. *Remedial Hygiene* is thus seen to be but a modification of *Preservative* or *General Hygiene.*

Why are not those things best adapted to preserve health, also best adapted to restore it? To us, it is one of the greatest mysteries of the ages that rational beings could ever have expected to restore health with anything other than the natural or normal agencies of health. Health is directly dependent on the primary act of organization, that of constructing or building up, from elemental materials of the blood, the organs by which function is performed. Materials that are not usable in this process have no business in the body under any circumstance.

There are certain fundamental conditions proper to the mental and physical well-being of man, and we must understand, as a matter of the strictest science, as well as of individual experience, that health is maintained or lost in exact proportion as these fundamental conditions are supplied or denied. This is one of the first important truths in reference to our physical organization which we must learn, if we are to have health on anything more than the haphazard basis commonly accepted. For, when the conditions of normal life are not fulfilled, it is inevitable that sickness ensue; when they are adequately fulfilled, health is equally inevitable.

How shall we determine our choice of materials and conditions for the care of the body in health and sickness? We must let the living organism answer this question for us. The human constitution is the final umpire before which all such questions must be arbitrated. Can the body use the materials in the production of tissue or in carrying on the functions of life? If the body cannot transform the material into living structure, it is valueless. But it is worse than valueless—if it is non-usable, it is poisonous, it is injurious, it occasions disease and death when introduced into the body.

The living organism has definite relations to everything in its environment—to certain things, a relation of affinity; to others a relation of antagonism. To those substances, influences and conditions that are opposed to the organic welfare, the body brings out its forces of defense in order that it may preserve its integrity. This defense, this resistance is wasteful of the powers of life and every indulgence in any poison, whether for "pleasure," as in swallowing coffee, tea, or alcohol, or in smoking or chewing tobacco, or for so-called medicinal purposes, weakens the powers of life by so much as the body must exert itself in resisting and expelling the poison. The resistance may be violent, as in acute poisoning; or it may be weak, but persistent, as in chronic poisoning, but in either event it is enervating and hurtful. It should be understood, in this connection, that whatever is hurtful to the body of man is also hurtful to his mind.

Health and the best means of promoting it cannot be studied in the sick room. The conditions and materials of health are best studied in the healthiest specimens. Whatever the body seeks and appropriates in a state of health is a hygienic factor; whatever it rejects and resists in a state of health is not a *hygienic* factor. If the body cannot make use of a substance in health, it is equally valueless in a state of disease. For, the relations of non-usable substances to the body are not changed in disease.

Why should a person be poisoned because he is sick? Is there any more reason why a sick person should be poisoned than there is why a well person should be poisoned? The idea of a peculiar health giving quality with which popular opinion invests drugs, is quite an erroneous one, and even professional notions of their antidotal quality, as related to *disease*, are false and certainly lack adequate scientific confirmation. Physiology affords us no knowledge of any power in the living organism by which it can manufacture either tissue or energy out of drug elements, or by which it can eliminate the causes of disease with such elements. On the contrary, the physiologist knows all too well, that drugs are only means whereby the system may be exhausted in a very unnecessary and wasteful manner. Any interference with the processes of life, in either health or disease, except by supplying appropriate elements for its use and proper conditions for appropriating them, is always and under all circumstances a serious mistake.

The chief materials and conditions concerned in vital processes are air, water, food, sunshine, temperature, exercise or activity, rest and sleep, cleanliness and wholesome mental and moral influences. The sum of the whole of these, when rightly used, is health. When any or all of them is abused, not used, or put to perverted or unphysiological use, disease results. *Preservative Hygiene,* that is, hygienic care of the well to the end that health may be maintained, is the correct employment of these factor-elements of normal living plus the persistent avoidance of abnormal elements or habits that we have foolishly, though, perhaps, ignorantly introduced into our modes of living.

When, in our manner of living, we violate, whether through ignorance or in spite of knowledge, certain organic laws, obedience to which alone can preserve health, we must inevitably suffer the necessary consequence of such violations. The function of *Hygiene* is to respect the laws of life and not to try to find means of circumventing their operations, nor to attempt to find means of erasing the effects of their violation while the violation is continued. We recognize no proffered medicinal indulgencies as valid or effective. Basic to the preservation of health is strict obedience to the laws of life in all of their relations. Only by obedience to the laws of life can we transmute into a song of gladness that moan of pain and wail of despair that goes up from the earth today.

In strictest accuracy, no man can break a law of nature. The professor who said that the man who steps off a tall building does not violate the law of gravity, he illustrates it, well expressed this fact. The same law produces different results under different conditions. The same law of gravity that carries a balloon upward under one set of conditions, brings it back to earth under another set of conditions; the same law of gravity that floats a ship under one set of conditions, sinks it under another set of conditions. The same law of chemical affinity that preserves a stick of dynamite under one set of conditions, explodes it under another set of conditions. So, the same laws of life that give us health under one set of conditions, give us disease under another set of conditions. In all of these instances, there is no change in the law, only changes in the conditions under which the law operates. If, then, we know the conditions for the production of health and the conditions for the production of disease, we may produce the one or the other as certainly as the chemist may produce and preserve a stick of dynamite or explode it. The choice is ours when we have the knowledge of the law and the conditions of its varied operations in the production of its varied results. Hereafter, then, when we speak of violations of the laws of life, it should be understood that this is merely a convenient phrase by which to indicate that wrong conditions of life are supplied the body.

We have no control over the laws of nature other than our ability to determine the results of their operations by supplying the different conditions required for the varied results of their operations. We can and we do control conditions under which laws operate. It is within our power to supply the conditions of health and to avoid the conditions of disease; it is equally within our power to supply the conditions of disease and deny the conditions of health. In saying this, it is not meant to imply that our power is absolute; nor, yet, that we now know all of the conditions of health and disease; nor is it meant to imply that the individual is not subject to social and environmental conditions that are not easily controlled by him. Fortunately, social and environmental conditions may often be escaped, while most of them may yet be socially controlled, so that in the future, as mankind becomes more enlightened, such evils will be gradually eliminated.

When we know the law and understand it, when we know how to obey and how to conform to it in every particular, when we know all of the conditions under which it operates to produce its many and varied results, then will it become a source of joy and of blessings rather than a stern, implacable and unsatisfying master. Obeying the law will become a hearty and enjoyable privilege and will provide us with fullness of life and superbness of health. The joys of the past will be eclipsed in that day when knowledge of the law and the conditions of its operations shall be the common property of everybody. This will bring joys, until then, untasted and unknown, joys before which the false joys of disobedience and indulgence will fade into nothingness.

I would emphasize that there are no substitutes for the hygienic factors upon which life and health depend. So old and so deeply ingrained is the drug superstition that it is very difficult to convince large numbers of otherwise intelligent people of the fallacy of the belief that drugs can be made to substitute for sensible eating, proper foods, pure water, fresh air, sunshine, rest, sleep, exercise, etc.—in short, for all of the natural or normal circumstances which we know to be necessary for the preservation of health. They persist in clinging to the wholly irrational belief that when pure food, or pure water, or fresh air, or sunshine are not available to them, drugs are proper substitutes therefor. I have previously emphasized that drugs cannot be used by the body, neither in health nor in disease. The use of drugs is based on age-old delusions that we should rapidly outgrow.

In the combined and systematic employment of all of the hygienic factors in harmony with physiological need and capacity, lies the way back to health. The use of these factors in disease must be modified to conform with the modified needs and capacities of the sick body. Here is precisely the line of demarkation between *general hygiene*, by the observance of which we seek to preserve the body in health, and *remedial hygiene*, or the natural means of restoring the body to health. We use the terms *modified* and *systematic* emphatically, because the *Hygienic* plan of caring for the sick consists in attending to health, to all of those matters concerned in the regular and ordinary production and maintenance of health, carefully graduating these to the changed conditions and needs of the sick organism, for it is the *Hygienic* position that only those materials and conditions can be of use to the body in illness, as in health, to which the body has a suitable relation.

The grand truth that both the acute and chronic sufferer is restored to health, after the cause of his suffering has been removed, by the self-same means, systematically and perseveringly applied, which are requisite for the preservation of health and continuance of life, must, sooner or later, be accepted by all mankind. This principle should appear to be, at least, normal and probable, even to the man in the street, when he first comes in contact with it. The scientifically trained man should realize its truth at once. Here is a principle that will serve mankind as a guiding rule, a compass by which to steer in the great sea of perplexity with which we are surrounded.

Hygienic care is the only radical and rational care that has ever been administered to the sick in any age of the world at any place. The time must come when all forms of disease will be cared for on the broad and infallible basis of *Hygienic* principles, for, when true principles are discovered, they are found to apply, not to one or two diseases only, nor to but one class of diseases, but to all diseases whatsoever. The same fundamental principle will apply throughout the whole catalogue of diseases. When rationally understood, *Natural Hygiene* is founded on physiological laws and must necessarily be the proper care of practically all diseased individuals and, in those cases where surgery is called upon for aid, must form the groundwork for the surgical procedure.

The first requirement of recovery of health is removal of all causes of impairment of health. It is as absurd to expect to restore health without removing the causes that have impaired it, as to attempt to sober up a drunk man while he continues to drink. While *Hygiene* strikes at the causes of disease and uproots the darling vices of the patient, and corrects those conditions to which the symptoms are due, the "curing" systems all toy with symptoms and seek to suppress these. This constitutes a fundamental difference between the two approaches to disease.

The air of our cities is filled with just about anything and everything that our bodies do not want, cannot use, and will probably work themselves to death trying to expel. Our water supplies are systematically drugged with a variety of chemicals, none of which should ever enter the body, our foods are processed, refined, adulterated, artificially flavored and colored, sprayed, produced on defective soils and treated in other ways that conspire to rob civilized man of adequate and suitable nutrient materials and that introduce poisons of various kinds into his body. Our cities are filled with noises and hubbub, our lives are filled with excitement and hurry, there is no peace, no calm, our very nights are turned into days of excitement and activity.

We habitually over eat, over work, indulge in sexual excesses, secure insufficient sleep, receive little or no sunshine, and over indulge in most of the good things of life. We are subject to worries, fears, anxieties, frustrations, inner conflicts, annoyances, irritations, jealousies, hatreds, domestic disharmonies, and infelicities, and to many other emotional over-irritations that help to impair the powers of life.

We are a nation of drug addicts—coffee, tea, chocolate, cocoa, alcohol, tobacco addicts. A veritable Niagara of poisoned "soft drinks" cascades down the American throat each day. Headache "remedies," constipation "cures," antacids for sour stomach, and many other drugs are used daily in great quantities by people who refuse to learn to live and eat to avoid suffering. They prefer to indulge and suppress the resulting symptoms to living intelligently and enjoying good health.

If we could accurately estimate the impairing influences of bad food, bad air, bad drink, too little, too much and improper exercise of the different bodily powers, of poisons of various kinds, of passional indulgencies, etc., we would know that our bodies are laboring at all times under a heavy load of abuse, which inevitably weakens and impairs every function of life. There is something else to do in life besides tinker with diet. Life is more than food. People are sick from bad habits of mind and body, and if they are to get well or to remain well, they must correct all of these habits.

All of these evils produce the same effect. Overwork produces a lowering of nerve energy—*enervation*. Fear, worry, inner conflict

and other emotional irritations produce enervation. Stimulation produces enervation. Overeating produces enervation. Sexual excesses
produce enervation. Lack of sleep produces enervation. Enervation
is the result of a mode of living—physical and mental—that uses up
nerve energy in excess of the power to recuperate or regenerate it
during the hours allotted to rest and repose.

Enervation lowers function throughout the body. Secretion and
excretion are checked. Nutrition is impaired and elimination is inhibited by enervation. Checked elimination results in a retention and
gradual accumulation of body waste—*metabolites*. This results in
poisoning by retained waste—*toxemia*. Toxemia is the universal,
basic cause of all disease. Toxemia is autogenerated and constant.
Wrong living produces enervation, enervation results in toxemia,
toxemia produces disease. The disease that develops will be in keeping with individual tendencies—*diathesis*.

Before recovery of health can occur, toxemia must be eliminated, nerve energy must be restored to normal and the mode of living
must be corrected. Doing all of this is removing cause. Failing to
do this, cause is not removed. If cause is not removed the patient
remains sick. Symptoms may be suppressed or palliated, organs may
be removed, crises may come and go, but the systemic toxemia remains to produce an ever recurring crop of new and old symptoms.
There is no health.

Previously, we have said that if we would eliminate we must
do it as nature does it. We cannot eliminate toxemia with "blood
purifiers." We cannot purify the blood by the use of enemas, co-
lonic irrigations, sweat baths, water drinking, juice drinking, and by
the use of the host of other forcing measures employed by the *curing*
professions. These measures are enervating and to substitute one
source of enervation for another is not a rational procedure. *Hygienists* reject as non-usable, ineffective and harmful, all treatments, substitutes and compromises.

Fasting (physiological rest) is nature's great scheme of elimination. In general more rest and sleep and less food and activity are
required for recovery. Nature, herself, enforces this rule in acute
disease and to a lesser extent in chronic disease. Mental and physical rest are not alone required for recuperation and conservation of
precious vital energies, but also for increased function by the organs

of elimination. By means of the principle of compensation (in order to increase activity on the one hand nature must decrease activity on the other), all energy saved by reducing or suspending one activity is available for increasing another.

There is a time to eat and a time not to eat; a time when the body needs and can appropriate food and a time when it cannot digest and assimilate the simplest of foods. It is necessary to know when to feed and when to fast a patient. It is possible to carry a fast too far; it is possible to break it prematurely. In the first instance the patient is damaged, in the second he fails to receive the legitimately expected results. Fasting, like feeding, must be graduated to the needs and abilities of the patient.

The second general requirement of recovery of health is that of supplying the normal requirements of health. After all enervating practices have been corrected and discontinued and rest and fasting have enabled the body to purify itself and recuperate its dissipated energies, building a state of vigorous, vital health can come only from the correct use of the elements of nature's own hygienic plan. As previously pointed out, if we would build, we must do it as nature builds—not with "tonics," stimulants (irritants), synthetic foods, and artificial measures, but by the rational use of the combined materials and influences that constitute the normal elements of life, or living.

We must tap the richest sources of vitality which nature possesses and turn these to valuable account. We must supply ourselves and our children with superior nutritive substances and these can come only from nature. Not to the chemist nor to the food manufacturer, must we go for superior nutrition, but to the original source of nutritive material. In nature's products are the requisites of superior nutrition.

We must supply ourselves and our children with sunshine and not with the rays from artificial lights—so-called sunlamps. The influence of the rays of the sun on human thoughts and actions are only less appreciable than those upon the growth of the melon vine, but because they affect man through the media of so many more relations, besides their direct effects, they are even more important to man than to the melon vine. In the complex organism of man glow the same solar fires that burn brightly in the melon vine and its luscious fruit.

We must supply ourselves and our children with appropriate exercise, an abundance of fresh air, with pure water, plenty of rest and sleep; we must avoid dissipating the energies of life with extremes of heat and cold in bathing; we must, in every way seek to conserve and not to dissipate the forces of life. Cleanliness is essential at all ages of life.

The influence of good morals on health is something with which every physician and every doctor, of whatever school of so-called healing, is well acquainted. All of us have observed how much better chance of life or of recovery from both acute and chronic states, one has whose "heart" is serenely fixed upon the good and the true. This may be said to be a sunshine of being by which every good man and woman is richly repaid for his or her righteous self-direction. All who sincerely cherish and cultivate the spirit of the good life reap a rich and abundant reward in health and strength, the kind of strength that enables one to endure and conquer.

The elimination of fear, worry, anxiety, jealousy, self-pity, inner conflicts, etc., is a negative factor. We must cultivate the positive virtues and qualities of love, cheer, hope, courage, friendship, poise, equilibrium or equanimity and good will. Our food tastes better when prepared by someone we love. The arrival of one deeply loved often brings renewed life to the dying. The loss of a loved one often occasions such a depression of the powers of life that death results. Browbeating and harsh treatment of patients, practices often indulged by physicians and nurses, often kill outright. Love and affection are essential to recovery.

Yet, how great is the number of patients who have sunk into their graves in both chronic and acute disease, amid the sweetest consolations of love, friendship and consanginuity, thus attesting the insufficiency of affection to preserve the object of its solicitude, when disconnected from the series of appropriate hygienic materials and influences that constitute the very foundation stones of life.

This brings us to an important feature of the *Hygienic System*: it is no one-method approach to the problems of health, disease and healing, but insists upon a total, an all-out approach to the many and complex problems of life and living. It is made up of many inter-dependent and concurrent means of care that collectively constitute preservative care in health and *remedial* care in illness. It is not a system of dieting, nor a "fasting cure," nor a "rest cure," nor a "sun cure," nor, yet, a "mind cure." No one element of *Hygiene* can ever represent the entire system. As a scientific fact, it is the whole of the hygienic materials and influences in their plenary combination and harmonious co-adaptation to the wants of the body that constitute the *remedial means of Natural Hygiene.* The ills of the patient are not to be remedied by fragments, but through the true relationship of all the elements of life in *organic unity.*

Tremendously important as is food, it is of value only in its physiological connections with air, water, sunshine, temperature, exercise or activity, rest and sleep, and the other elements of nature's hygienic plan. When once, by *Hygienic* means, the body has been freed of its load of toxins, its nerve energy has been restored to normal, elimination has been reestablished and assimilative powers have been restored, there follows a gradual return to vigorous health. Until this has been done, the best of diets cannot and will not give desired results. The same fact is equally true of all the other factor-elements of the *Hygienic System.* Only by the rational use of the combined materials and conditions that constitute the *Hygienic System* can the enfeebled organism be restored to strength and vigor. Only by first removing the causes of enfeeblement and, then supplying rest, sleep, food, of the proper kind, exercise, air, water, sunshine and healthful mental and moral influences can we hope to restore integrity of structure and efficiency of function to the sick.

All of these hygienic elements are to be supplied the sick organism in harmony with its needs and capacities under prevailing conditions and not according to any arbitrary or laboratory standard. The amount of food given the patient must always be graduated in proportion to his strength. The more feeble his body, the less digestive power he has, hence stuffing the sick on "rich" viands, under the supposition that they need so much food, or that "plenty of good nourishing food" will build them up, is a common but fallacious practice. It is usually best to withhold food until the power to digest has been restored.

What was known as the *analeptic* treatment, one that is most often resorted to in illness and during convalescence, came into use in the care of tubercular patients about a hundred years ago and has killed many thousands of tubercular patients since. An "analeptic" is a "restorative" a "strengthener." Analeptic treatment was intended to restore strength. It was made up of "nourishing" foods and "tonics." This treatment of the tubercular and convalescent is still in vogue in medical circles. Under the reign of the fallacy that food gives strength, patients are not only encouraged and coerced into eating far more food than they have the ability to utilize, they are actually, in many instances, forcibly fed. Coercion and forced feeding violate every psychological need of good digestion, besides feeding when the physiological requirements of good digestion are lacking.

The principle of graduating the employment of hygienic factors to the needs and abilities of the patient applies to the employment of exercise, sunshine, rest and all other hygienic factors. It never helps the patient to overdo any good thing; it never achieves full results to stop short of enough. Wholesome food taken in excess becomes a dissipation. Too much exercise is exhausting. Too much sunshine is very enervating.

It will now be seen that *Hygiene* embraces and seeks to embrace truths in nature and seeks to learn their proper application to the preservation and restoration of health. Thus it embodies a correct science and art of care of both the well and the sick. It relies, therefore, upon no favorable accident to result from maneuvering the body with materials and conditions that have no normal relations to life. It turns physiology to the use of body care and is exultant at the range of means to it from this source, which are competent to secure the highest results.

The effects of such a plan of care are entirely in the direction of natural growth and of physiological development and are, consequently, of a permanent character. Its influences are manifested throughout all of the physiological channels and especially in every function, the defective action of which gives rise to morbid symptoms. *Hygiene* is quite distinct from any other plan of care that has ever been devised and does not mix with any of the therapeutic schemes in vogue, or that have been in vogue.

Every person who has been long an invalid feels to the very core of his being the want of the remedial plan here proposed; and every such one will regard it as covering unoccupied ground, as supplying the most pressing and indispensable needs, and furnishing the most important, but sadly neglected desideratum in the care of the sick. *Hygiene* is manifestly based on principles that command the respect and allegiance of the thoughtful and candid, because of its foundation in physiological law.